MISSION COLLEGE
LIBRARY

799

Expert Praise for the Family Guide to ... al Heal...

"Comprehensive, ... nd ... Sorts out fact from fan... ...m a lucid, interesting style."

—STEPHEN BRUNTON, M.D.
Clinical Professor
Department of Family Medicine
University of California Irvine

"Superbly written and understandable by those we wish to help—our patients and their families."

—EDWIN C. CADMAN, M.D.
Ensign Professor and Chairman
Department of Internal Medicine
Yale University School of Medicine

"A must for every household where there are concerns about safe use of medications ... An ideal way to clarify and supplement the information provided by your health care provider."

—JACK M. ROSENBERG, Pharm.D., Ph.D.
Professor of Clinical Pharmacy and
   Pharmacology
Director, Division of Pharmacy Practice
Arnold & Marie Schwartz College of
   Pharmacy and Health Sciences
Long Island University

*Please turn the page
for more reviews....*

MISSION COLLEGE
LIBRARY
Expert Advice for the PDR®
Family Guide Series of Personal
Health Handbooks

"As individuals increasingly empower themselves in a variety of areas in our society, so too are they requiring more information and input into their own medical care decisions. . . . A great resource for the patient in his or her dialogue with the physician."

—JOSEPH R. CRUSE, M.D.
Founding Medical Director
The Betty Ford Center

"An excellent supplement to the education that should occur during every health visit ... Allows people to find answers when and where they need them—any time of day or night in their own home."

—BARBARA P. YAWN, M.D., M.S.
Associate Professor of Clinical Family
Medicine and Community Health
University of Minnesota

"The premier professional drug reference guide now gives consumers their best guide to medical problems and the medications prescribed for them. . . . Clear, readable, comprehensive."
—BARRIE R. CASSILETH, Ph.D.
   Adjunct Professor
   University of North Carolina
      and Duke University Medical Center

"A valuable and timely adjunct in this age of consumer education, patient rights, and quality health care for all."
—ROBERTA S. ABRUZZESE, Ed.D., R.N.,
   F.A.A.N.
   Editor, *Decubitus: The Journal of Skin Ulcers*

"The *Physician's Desk Reference* (PDR®) has been rewritten in language the average mortal can understand."
            —Associated Press

Published by Ballantine Books:

THE PDR® FAMILY GUIDE TO OVER-THE-COUNTER
    DRUGS™
THE PDR® FAMILY GUIDE ENCYCLOPEDIA OF
    MEDICAL CARE™
THE PDR® FAMILY GUIDE TO COMMON
    AILMENTS™
THE PDR® FAMILY GUIDE TO NATURAL MEDICINES
    AND HEALING THERAPIES™
THE PDR® FAMILY GUIDE TO NUTRITIONAL
    SUPPLEMENTS™

Books published by The Ballantine Publishing Group
are available at quantity discounts on bulk purchases
for premium, educational, fund-raising, and special
sales use. For details, please call 1-800-733-3000.

THE PDR®
FAMILY GUIDE

TO NUTRITIONAL SUPPLEMENTS™

BALLANTINE BOOKS • NEW YORK

Sale of this book without a front cover may be unauthorized. If this book is coverless, it may have been reported to the publisher as "unsold or destroyed" and neither the author nor the publisher may have received payment for it.

A Ballantine Book
Published by The Ballantine Publishing Group
Copyright © 2001 by Medical Economics Company, Inc.

All rights reserved under International and Pan-American Copyright Conventions. Published in the United States by The Ballantine Publishing Group, a division of Random House, Inc., New York, and simultaneously in Canada by Random House of Canada Limited, Toronto.

None of the content of this publication may be reproduced, stored in a retrieval system, or transmitted in any form or by any means (electronic, mechanical, photocopying, recording, or otherwise) without prior written permission of Medical Economics Company, Inc., Five Paragon Drive, Montvale, N.J. 07645.

Ballantine is a registered trademark and the Ballantine colophon is a trademark of Random House, Inc.

www.ballantinebooks.com

ISBN 0-345-43376-9

Manufactured in the United States of America

First Edition: December 2001

10 9 8 7 6 5 4 3 2 1

PHYSICIANS' DESK REFERENCE®, PDR®, Pocket PDR®, The PDR® Family Guide to Prescription Drugs®, The PDR® Family Guide to Women's Health and Prescription Drugs®, and The PDR® Family Guide to Nutrition and Health® are registered trademarks used herein under license. PDR for Ophthalmic Medicines™, PDR for Nonprescription Drugs and Dietary Supplements™, PDR Companion Guide™, PDR Pharmacopoeia™ Pocket Dosing Guide, PDR® for Herbal Medicines™, PDR® for Nutritional Supplements™, PDR® Medical Dictionary™, PDR® Nurse's Drug Handbook™, PDR® Nurse's Dictionary™, The PDR® Family Guide Encyclopedia of Medical Care™, The PDR® Family Guide to Natural Medicines and Healing Therapies™, The PDR® Family Guide to Common Ailments™, The PDR® Family Guide to Over-the-Counter Drugs™, The PDR® Family Guide to Nutritional Supplements™, and PDR® Electronic Library™ are trademarks used herein under license.

Officers of Thomson Healthcare: *Chief Executive Officer:* Michael Tansey; *Chief Operating Officer:* Richard Noble; *Chief Financial Officer and Executive Vice President, Finance:* Paul Hilger; *Executive Vice President, Directory Services:* Paul Walsh; *Senior Vice President, Planning and Business Development:* William Gole; *Vice President, Human Resources:* Pamela M. Bilash

Contents

CONTENTS

The PDR® Family Guide to Nutritional Supplements™

Contributors and Consultants

Editor-in-Chief: David W. Sifton

Medical Advisors: Richard Galbraith, M.D., Ph.D., Professor of Medicine, the University of Vermont College of Medicine; Naomi K. Fukagawa, M.D., Ph.D., Associate Professor of Medicine, the University of Vermont College of Medicine

Senior Associate Editors: Janette V. Carlucci; Lori Murray

Assistant Editor: Gwynned L. Kelly

Writers: Nancy K. Bannon; Brenda L. Becker; Paul L. Cerrato; Kris Hallam; Ami Havens; Judith K. Ludwig, Ph.D.; Lisa A. Maher; Cynthia H. Starr, M.S., R.Ph.; Marissa J. Ventura

Medical Economics Company

Executive Vice President, Directory Services: Paul Walsh

Vice President, Clinical Communications and New Business Development: Mukesh Mehta, R.Ph.

Vice President, Sales and Marketing: Dikran N. Barsamian

Director of Trade Sales: Bill Gaffney

Publisher's Note

The PDR® Family Guide to Nutritional Supplements™ is the product of an extensive review of the relevant literature. Nevertheless, it's important to remember that it merely summarizes and synthesizes key data from the underlying reports, and of necessity includes neither every published report nor every recorded fact. Observations regarding the effectiveness of the nutritional supplements discussed in this book are based on the preponderance of current evidence and are neither conclusive nor final. The publisher does not warrant that a nutritional supplement will provide any of the effects claimed for it. Likewise, the publisher does not guarantee that every possible hazard, adverse effect, contraindication, precaution, or consequence of overdose is included in the summaries presented here. All dosage recommendations cited in the text are those of the supplement's suppliers and other advocates, and not those of the publisher. The publisher has performed no independent verification of the data reported herein, and expressly disclaims responsibility for any error. All information is presented without guarantees by the authors, consultants, and publisher, who disclaim all liability in connection with its use.

It should be understood that by making this material available, the publisher is not advocating the use of any substance described herein. Inclusion of a substance does not signify an endorsement by the publisher; absence of a substance does not imply rejection. Please remember that in the United States, nutritional supplements and herbal products must be in compliance with the Dietary Supplement Health and Education Act of 1994, which stipulates that they may not be marketed for the diagnosis, treatment, cure, or prevention of any disease. The profiles in this book do not discuss claims made for any specific proprietary dietary supplement. They merely report general findings on generic nutrients and botanicals.

This book is intended only as a reference for use in an ongoing partnership between doctor and patient in the comprehensive management of the patient's health. It is not a substitute for a doctor's professional judgment, and it serves only as a guide to the many options and issues that may bear discussion. All readers are urged to consult with a physician before undertaking any form of self-diagnosis or self-treatment with nutritional, herbal, and other over-the-counter remedies.

Foreword:
The Promises and Pitfalls
of Dietary Supplements

There's no question about it: Better food is good medicine. As scientists learn more and more about the potent nutrients that lace our everyday diet, they're discovering unsuspected benefits that sometimes rival the impact of prescription drugs.

Welcome to the exciting new world of "designer foods" and "nutraceuticals." Here you'll find a host of natural substances that promise to boost immunity, fend off cancer, sharpen memory, and lift depression. There are "phytosterols" to bring down your cholesterol, "probiotics" to improve your digestion, and "phyto-estrogens" to relieve the symptoms of menopause. A variety of oils, acids, and enzymes offer protection for your heart. And to build muscle and renew energy, a staggering array of "ergogenic aids" await you with a bevy of alluring claims.

But note this carefully: Too often in the world of nutritional supplements, the operative word is "claim." While the evidence in favor of certain substances continues to mount, the effectiveness of others remains totally unverified. Every product has an appealing theoretical rationale, but for many, that's where the story ends. Either tests have failed to detect any benefit or—more often than not—no reliable tests have been conducted.

Products that haven't undergone adequate testing pose an especially difficult dilemma. On one hand, claims made for such products could be totally genuine. On the other, they might be completely bogus. Without the kind of exhaustive clinical trials that medical authorities and smart consumers demand today, it's impossible to tell—and no one can say for certain whether such products are worth trying or not.

Because many nutritional supplements hold truly great promise, this book endeavors to steer a middle course, describing each product's potential benefits whether conclusively proven or not, but clearly distinguishing between claims that scientists consider valid and those that are still regarded as theoretical. When a substance flat-out doesn't work, we'll tell you. Most of the time, however, you'll find that the scientific evidence remains in limbo—neither conclusively *pro* nor absolutely *con*.

In the end, it's up to you and your doctor to decide what's worth a try. But choose thoughtfully, and remember that in the realm of nutritional supplements it's especially important for the buyer to beware. In this book, we've summarized special cautions to take with each specific supplement. No matter what the product, however, always keep the following general do's and don'ts in mind.

Do choose a supplier you trust

Nutritional supplements are not subject to regulation by the U.S. Food and Drug Administration, so they're not routinely checked for purity and potency. When private consumer watchdog groups do a spot check, they sometimes find that the products contain little or none of the active ingredients they claim.

Worse yet, when buying from an unreliable source, you also run the risk of contamination. In the late 1980s, contaminated batches of the usually harmless amino acid tryptophan killed more than 30 people. Even a seemingly innocuous product such as bone meal may contain unhealthy levels of lead, and supplements refined from animal sources, such as desiccated liver, could be laced with growth hormones and antibiotics. When choosing any supplement, stick with established manufacturers that have a reputable name.

Don't rely on supplements to replace existing therapy

Although there's little doubt that certain nutritional supplements can boost immune function, protect the heart, and relieve a wide variety of specific ailments, in most cases they work best as an adjunct to traditional treatments. For instance, although coenzyme Q10 may help boost cardiac function, patients with congestive heart failure would be in for an unpleasant surprise if they attempted to use it in place of their regular prescription medication. Likewise, someone with HIV may benefit from certain supplements, but it would be suicide to use them *instead of* regular AIDS drugs.

Do avoid virtually all supplements during pregnancy

Aside from a handful of vitamins—such as folic acid—that are known to be important during pregnancy, virtually no dietary supplements have been tested for safety when used during this critical period. Taken in reasonable amounts, many are probably harmless—but we don't know this for sure. Since anyone can live without these supplements for a matter of months, there's no reason to expose the baby to even the slight possibility of risk that a supplement may harbor.

Don't assume that if a little is good, a lot is better

Even supplements as common as vitamins A and D can be poisonous in large doses. Phosphorus is essential for healthy bones, but too much can actually promote bone loss. Likewise, amino acids, the building blocks of protein, are needed to maintain all the body's tissues, but excessive amounts won't build extra muscle and could overburden the kidneys and liver, doing more harm than good. And while many researchers think that small amounts of phytoestrogen might protect against cancer, they're beginning to suspect that large doses could have the opposite effect.

The key is balance. When using supplements, remember that the goal is to *fine-tune* your body chemistry, not reorganize it. Nutrients interact in unexpected ways, so that an increase in one may demand a compensatory increase in another. Similarly, hormones affect each other in complex ways that can lead to unforeseen consequences. Use moderation, and be careful to follow your doctor's recommendations.

Do remember that "natural" isn't necessarily safe

Some of history's most celebrated poisons—hemlock, nightshade, and wormwood—are entirely natural. Natural substances such as bee pollen and bee propolis can harbor unpleasant natural contaminants. And, as we've seen, natural everyday nutrients may have unwanted side effects when taken in unnatural amounts.

In any event, many "natural" products are distinctly artificial. Some are synthetic versions of the real thing. Others are so highly refined that they act more like drugs than like food—possibly with greater benefits, but also with greater risks. Never assume a product is benign just because it's labeled "natural."

Don't go to the health food store instead of a doctor

Yes, the right supplements may relieve specific ailments, but first you need to be certain of the problem. The human body is so complex that even doctors have trouble diagnosing many ailments. And lacking the necessary knowledge and tests, it's a sure thing that you won't be able to diagnose yourself. If you try, it's all too likely that you'll wind up taking the wrong supplement for the wrong reason, while your underlying condition gets worse.

On the other hand, once you know what's wrong, don't hesitate to take full advantage of what nutritional science has revealed. The right nutrients, in the right amounts, really can improve your health and fend off disease. Some of the supplements described in this book may be a disappointment—and some may be virtually useless—but many others can be expected to deliver on their promise. There's no reason to delay. Get to work with your doctor to get the most out of them and the rest of your diet.

Alginates

Why People Take Them

Derived from brown seaweeds, these substances are a surprisingly common part of the American diet. The food industry uses them as a thickening, stabilizing, or gelling agent in foods such as ice cream, pudding, and salad dressings. As food additives, they are rated "generally recognized as safe" by the U.S. Food and Drug Administration.

In the health care industry, dentists use Alginates to create dental impressions. Alginates are also reportedly useful for removing toxins such as lead from the body. And, for some time, these compounds have been used as wound dressings because of their ability to absorb excess fluid from the wound while keeping the wound itself moist. (But whether this type of dressing actually promotes healing is a subject of continued debate.)

As medicines, Alginates are used primarily for relief of indigestion and heartburn, taken alone or in combination with antacids. There is some evidence to support their value as a heartburn remedy. At least one clinical study has found that an Alginate liquid reduced the number of attacks of acid backflow (reflux) that leads to heartburn. (But the study also found that, when reflux did occur, the Alginate did not shorten its duration.)

Another study found greater improvement in symptoms of gastroesophageal reflux disease (GERD) among people treated with Alginate than among those treated with the prescription drug Propulsid (a heartburn remedy that was recently taken off the market due to potentially dangerous interactions with other drugs). However, a third study found that treatment with yet another prescription drug—namely, omeprazole (Prilosec)—was more effective in relieving symptoms of GERD than an antacid/Alginate combination.

A variety of other claims have been made for Alginates. They are being investigated as a possible cancer preventive. They are being studied for their role in treating diabetes, stimulating the growth of human skin cells, and immobilizing cells for transplantation purposes. The possibility that they can boost the immune system is also being examined. To date, however, none of these potential benefits has been conclusively verified.

What They Are; How They Work

Alginates are a form of indigestible polysaccharide (fiber). There are various types, all derived from the salts of alginic acid; they include ammonium alginate, calcium alginate, potassium alginate, and sodium alginate.

Their "healing power" comes from their ability to absorb fluids and to form a gel. In the treatment of gastroesophageal reflux, for example, Alginates are believed to form a foamlike layer that floats on the surface of gastric contents in the stomach and prevents the backflow of these contents into the esophagus.

Avoid if . . .
Don't take Alginates if you have an allergy to seaweed or are sensitive to iodine.

Special Cautions
In one study, Alginates were found to cause constipation, digestive difficulties, and weight gain. However, such problems are rare.

Possible Drug Interactions
Alginates may decrease intestinal absorption. For example, they could affect the absorption of other treatments for gastroesophageal reflux disorder such as ranitidine (Tritec, Zantac) or cimetidine (Tagamet). If you're taking these or any other drugs, it's best to check with your doctor before taking Alginates.

Special Information if You Are Pregnant or Breast-feeding
Although there's no reason to suspect a problem, the effect of Alginates on a developing baby has not been studied. It's wise to check with your doctor before taking this or any other supplement while pregnant or breast-feeding.

Available Preparations and Dosage
Alginates are available in tablet, capsule, powder, and liquid form. Over-the-counter tablets containing Alginates are usually found in combinations with antacids.

Clinical studies involving liquid Alginate typically used doses ranging from 10 to 20 milliliters. The recommended dose for an antacid/Alginate tablet is two tablets containing 200 milligrams of alginic acid.

Overdosage
No information on overdosage is available.

Androstenedione

Why People Take It
With a surge of publicity over the use of Androstene-dione (Andro) by popular athletes such as home run king Mark McGwire, sales of this trendy over-the-counter supplement have soared. Promoters of Andro claim that it boosts testosterone levels—an appealing effect for athletes and bodybuilders who want increased muscle mass and athletic endurance. There are also reports that it enhances the sex drive and sexual performance.

However, the popularity of Andro, especially among teenage athletes, has set off alarms in the medical community. Concern over the safety of this hormonal precursor has prompted increased scientific investigation and revealed some decidedly unwanted effects. While not illegal, the substance is now banned by the International Olympic Committee, the National Football League, the National Basketball Association, and the National Collegiate Athletic Association for use by their athletes. Physicians argue that it is a powerful steroid and warn that its effects, especially in the long term, are not known and could have a negative impact on health. Consequently, there are groups working to have it banned completely by the U.S. Food and Drug Administration.

Bottom line: This product delivers results, but possibly more than you bargained for. Until more is known about the health risks associated with Androstenedione, use it only with your doctor's advice.

What It Is; How It Works

Androstenedione is a naturally occurring hormone precursor produced primarily in the testes of men. The body converts Androstenedione into the male sex hormone testosterone, which is responsible for male sexual characteristics such as facial hair, lower voice, and larger muscles. It is also produced in smaller amounts by the adrenal glands of both men and women. Testosterone is responsible for muscle building and is part of a healthy hormonal balance in both sexes.

Promoters of synthetic over-the-counter Andro insist that it is safe and that oral doses are converted directly to boost testosterone levels in the bloodstream, resulting in increased muscle strength and mass, and endurance. However, the evidence is mixed. One study did show that 300 milligrams of Andro increased testosterone levels in men, though it found the effect short-lived—no more than three hours—because testosterone breaks down quickly in the body, making high frequent dosing necessary for sustained results. But another study that measured blood levels of testosterone and muscle strength and mass concluded that 300 milligrams of

Andro did *not* boost testosterone levels in males or produce the muscle-building results that promoters promise.

Both research teams agreed, however, on one little-advertised effect: Regardless of its impact on testosterone, Androstenedione taken by men is converted into estradiol, a powerful female hormone. Both studies showed an increase in blood estrogen levels in the men who took Andro. This may account for several unwelcome side effects, including breast enlargement and lowered "good cholesterol" in some Andro users, in addition to an increased risk of liver problems and pancreatic cancer.

Other questions loom over the safety and efficacy of Androstenedione. Doctors don't know whether taking excessive amounts of the supplement orally interferes with the production or effects of naturally occurring testosterone. In addition, there's concern about the quality, purity, and stability of over-the-counter Androstenedione, since dietary supplements are largely unregulated.

Avoid if . . .

Women and children under the age of 18 should not take Androstenedione. Substances that work like steroids are known to stunt growth in children, and women may develop decreased breast size, deepened voice, facial hair growth, and menstrual irregularities. Men should avoid Andro if they have prostate cancer or an elevated PSA (prostate-specific androgen) level. Increased testosterone levels are associated with a greater risk of this cancer. Do not take Andro if you have a family history of any hormone-related cancer.

Special Cautions

Treatment with some forms of testosterone can cause liver damage, and may lead to water retention and swelling in people with kidney, liver, or heart disease. If you have one of these conditions, check with your doctor before using Andro. Also consult your doctor if you have diabetes or any serious psychological condition. Use Andro with caution if you have acne; it can make this condition worse.

Possible Drug Interactions

Do not use Androstenedione in combination with steroids or any other kind of hormone therapy. Such combinations increase the likelihood of side effects.

Special Information if You Are Pregnant or Breast-Feeding

All women should avoid Androstenedione, and that's doubly true for those who are pregnant or breast-feeding. Its potential hormonal effects could harm a developing baby.

Available Preparations and Dosage

Androstenedione is available in capsules, sublingual tablets, and sprays in strengths ranging from 50 milligrams to 250 milligrams. Most manufacturers recommend taking from 50 milligrams to 300 milligrams prior to exercise. Andro use should be cycled: if you take Andro for four to six weeks, follow it with a two-week break.

Overdosage

There's no information on Andro overdose, but an extreme overdose of testosterone has been implicated in a case of stroke.

Arabinogalactan

Why People Take It

Advocates of Arabinogalactan (also known as galacto-arabinan and larch gum) claim that it rivals the popular herb echinacea in its positive effects on the immune system. Arabinogalactan is said to help fight off infection two ways. First, it is thought to promote the growth of beneficial bacteria in the gut. Second, it is said to stimulate the activity of the body's natural killer (NK) cells, agents of the immune system that attack and destroy certain types of cancer cells and cells infected by viruses. Its ability to actually fend off disease has not, however, been tested in any sort of major clinical trial.

What It Is; How It Works

Arabinogalactan is a naturally occurring carbohydrate found in many common foods, including carrots, lettuce, tomatoes, spinach, radishes, corn, wheat, red wine, sorghum, and coconut. (Not surprisingly, it's also one of the active ingredients in echinacea.) Commercially produced Arabinogalactan is obtained from the sap of larch trees. Approved for use as a food additive by the FDA in the 1960s, Arabinogalactan is often used as a stabilizer, thickener, and texturizer in such products as nonnutritive sweeteners, flavor bases, and pudding mixes.

Evidence suggests that consuming Arabinogalactan supports the growth of the beneficial bacteria—such as *Lactobacillus acidophilus* and *Bifidobacterium bifidum*—that live in the human body and help promote good gastrointestinal health while increasing resistance to infections. (See separate entries.) There's some evidence that friendly bacteria may also normalize hormone levels, reduce cholesterol levels, and protect against some forms of cancer.

Experimental studies also indicate that Arabinogalactan may help inhibit bacteria from attaching to cells, slow the spread of tumor cells to the liver, and dramatically increase the activity of immune cells that destroy foreign invaders and cancer cells.

Avoid if . . .
There are no known reasons to avoid this supplement.

Special Cautions
No side effects have been reported.

Possible Drug Interactions
No interactions are known.

Special Information if You Are Pregnant or Breast-Feeding
This common food additive has been deemed safe for pregnant and breast-feeding women.

Available Preparations and Dosage
No standard dosage has been established. However, human studies conducted at several major U.S. universities found increased immune cell growth with a daily dose of 1.5 grams of Arabinogalactan.

Overdosage
No information on overdose is available.

Arginine

Why People Take It
Scientists discovered this amino acid—one of the raw materials of human protein—more than a century ago, but only recently has it become a popular dietary supplement. It is now being promoted as the "natural alternative to Viagra," a cure for erectile dysfunction. It has also been advertised as a natural remedy for other effects of aging if taken in doses larger than the body can produce. These sometimes extravagant claims remain largely un-

proven. In particular, Arginine's effect on erectile dysfunction is questionable. It has been shown to be of some benefit in tests on rats, but there have been no conclusive trials in humans.

Claims have also been made for Arginine as a tumor retardant and immune system stimulant, beneficial to those suffering from AIDS and other diseases that suppress the immune system. And several recent scientific studies suggest that Arginine may play a role in heart attack prevention by blocking the formation of plaque in arteries, widening blood vessels, and helping to prevent platelets from forming clots that block arteries.

Because Arginine promotes the production of growth hormone, some bodybuilders take it in the belief that it will aid in the development of muscle bulk. Many experts, however, warn against adult use of growth hormone—or substances such as Arginine that stimulate its release.

What It Is; How It Works

Arginine is classified as a "nonessential" amino acid because, if it's lacking in the diet, the body can usually manufacture the amount it needs. During periods of growth, healing, or stress, however, the body may not be able to keep up with demand, and dietary sources become essential. Arginine is available in meat and dairy products, as well as cereals, whole wheat, brown rice, nuts, beans, and raisins.

In addition to its role in protein synthesis and production of growth hormone, Arginine contributes to immune cell maintenance, and makes up a significant percentage of collagen, one of the major building blocks of cartilage and bone. It also appears naturally in seminal fluid, suggesting to some proponents that it may be a factor in sexual maturity, aiding sperm production and motility. This theoretical impact on male fertility adds to its appeal as a potential remedy for sexual dysfunction.

The body requires Arginine for the production of nitric oxide, a compound whose importance to health has only recently been recognized. Nitric oxide is one of the factors that control dilation of the blood vessels, and it may play a role in discouraging the circulatory disorders that often come with advancing age. Nitric oxide was named Molecule of the Year in 1993 by the journal *Science*, and the scientists who discovered its cardiovascular benefits received the Nobel Prize for Physiology in 1998.

The effect of nitric oxide on blood vessels may help some people with high blood pressure. It's also the basis for claims that Arginine can relieve erectile dysfunction. And a shortage of nitric oxide is known to accompany at least one other medical problem: interstitial cystitis, a painful inflammation of the bladder. Studies indicate that supplemental Arginine raises nitric oxide levels and can relax bladder muscle spasms to help control the pain for some sufferers.

The body converts some of its Arginine into ornithine, another important amino acid (see separate entry). Ornithine is necessary for proper immune system and liver function, helps rid the body of ammonia, and aids in liver regeneration.

Avoid if . . .

Children should not be given Arginine supplements due to this amino acid's impact on growth hormone levels. For the same reason, it should be avoided during pregnancy and breast-feeding. Arginine supplements may reactivate latent herpes virus infections (both genital herpes and cold sores); so if you have herpes it's wise to avoid them.

Special Cautions

Growth hormone and substances that promote its release, such as Arginine, can aggravate diabetes; diabetics should use them only under their doctor's supervision. Arginine may worsen some types of psychosis. Some critics charge that, while Arginine may retard the growth of some types of tumors, it seems to promote the growth of others.

Possible Drug Interactions

Do not take Arginine supplements with drugs that dilate the blood vessels, such as nitroglycerine or Viagra.

Special Information if You Are Pregnant or Breast-feeding

Because this amino acid activates growth hormone release, it's best to avoid Arginine supplements while pregnant or nursing.

Available Preparations and Dosage

Arginine is available as L-arginine (levo-rotatory form), which is produced by a fermentation process that separates it from other amino acids. It is also sold as ADNO (arginine-derived nitric oxide), and can be purchased in capsules combined with ornithine.

Manufacturers typically suggest daily dosages of 2 grams to improve male fertility and sexual performance, and 3 to 4 grams for the growth hormone effect. It is also available in some diet bars.

Overdosage
Large doses of Arginine may cause diarrhea, nausea, and, rarely, dizziness.

Arginine Pyroglutamate

Why People Take It
A modified form of the amino acid arginine (see separate entry), this nutritional supplement is used primarily by bodybuilders and people attempting to preserve their youth. Its popularity is based on the fact that, like arginine, it stimulates the release of human growth hormone. Enthusiasts believe this hormone can build muscle mass, improve endurance, and stave off old age. Unfortunately, there's scant evidence to support this view.

Arginine Pyroglutamate suffuses brain tissue more readily than regular arginine, so researchers have also been testing it as a treatment for cognitive dysfunction related to senility and alcoholism. To date, the results have been disappointing.

What It Is; How It Works

Arginine is one of the "nonessential" amino acids that the body can usually manufacture for itself when dietary supplies are insufficient. Most people don't need arginine supplements to prevent a deficiency. Extra supplies become necessary only under conditions of extreme physical stress, such as major injury, surgery, or infection, when the body can't keep up with demand.

Arginine plays a variety of important roles. It builds protein, supports immune cells, and provides raw material for the production of nitric oxide, a natural tonic for the heart and blood vessels. It promotes the production of several hormones, including insulin, prolactin, and human growth hormone, and it's a key ingredient of collagen, one of the major building blocks of cartilage and bone. Because some arginine is converted into the amino acid ornithine (see separate entry), which helps to rid the body of ammonia and aids in liver regeneration, it also supports healthy liver function. Arginine Pyroglutamate is, in fact, often marketed in combination with ornithine, despite the fact that there is little to be gained from such a combination.

Avoid if . . .

Because Arginine Pyroglutamate may increase levels of human growth hormone, it is not recommended for children and adolescents, who are still growing and, presumably, producing all the growth hormone they need. Its impact on growth hormone also makes it a bad choice during pregnancy and breast-feeding, and because some experts fear that growth hormone may promote the

growth of certain types of tumors, Arginine Pyroglutamate should also be avoided by anyone with a history of
or high risk for cancer.

Special Cautions

Due to the effect of arginine on insulin secretion, Arginine Pyroglutamate may not be appropriate for people
with diabetes. Arginine supplements have also been
known to trigger herpes outbreaks in infected individuals, and should be completely avoided by anyone
with brain or ocular herpes. Arginine may also worsen
schizophrenia.

Possible Drug Interactions

Arginine Pyroglutamate can dramatically reduce the effectiveness of barbiturates and some other sedatives used
in anesthesia. If you're taking Arginine Pyroglutamate,
check with your doctor before taking any drugs that affect the central nervous system.

Because arginine promotes dilated blood vessels, it's
wise to avoid combining arginine products and prescription drugs with a similar effect, including nitroglycerin,
Viagra, and some blood pressure medications. Avoid supplements of the amino acid lysine as well, since it cancels
some of arginine's effects.

Special Information if You Are Pregnant or Breast-feeding

Due to its stimulating effect on growth hormone, Arginine Pyroglutamate is not recommended during pregnancy or breast-feeding.

Available Preparations and Dosage

Arginine Pyroglutamate is available in tablet and capsule form, typically in strengths of 400 milligrams. Although there are no established dosages for this supplement, suppliers recommend between 2 and 8 tablets daily.

Overdosage

Even large doses of amino acids are generally nontoxic. However, excessive doses of arginine have been reported to cause diarrhea, nausea, and dizziness.

Aspartic Acid

Why People Take It

A beneficiary of the fitness craze, Aspartic Acid is one of the many amino acid compounds that bodybuilders take to improve performance, increase stamina, and minimize postexercise fatigue.

Some proponents also claim that Aspartic Acid helps promote mental alertness and suggest that it can combat chronic fatigue, depression, heart failure, irregular heartbeat, infertility, and toxemia. However, more clinical studies are needed to determine precisely what role, if any, Aspartic Acid should play as a dietary supplement for regular use.

What It Is; How It Works

Also known as aminosuccinic acid, asparagic acid, asparaginic acid, and aspartate, Aspartic Acid is one of the "nonessential" amino acids that the body can manufacture if they're lacking in the diet. Few Americans are likely to suffer a dietary deficiency of this amino acid, since it's found in a wide variety of animals and plants, including sugarcane, sugar beets, molasses, brewer's yeast, whole grains, dairy products, eggs, meat, fish, nuts, seeds, and beans.

Aspartic Acid plays an important role in carbohydrate metabolism and protein metabolism. It helps reduce blood ammonia levels after exercise—thus lessening fatigue—and serves as a carrier molecule for the transport of magnesium and potassium in your cells. By combining with other amino acids to form molecules that absorb toxins and remove them from the bloodstream, Aspartic Acid may help protect the liver and aid cell function. It's also involved in the production of DNA and RNA, the compounds that carry and transmit the genetic code.

Advocates of Aspartic Acid have proposed it as a treatment for depression because it is one of the major excitatory (stimulating) chemical messengers in the brain. Aspartic Acid levels are frequently decreased in people with unipolar depression and brain atrophy, and may be increased in those with seizures and strokes.

Aspartic Acid is the key raw material from which aspartame, the low-calorie artificial sweetener, is manufactured. Perhaps not coincidentally, some researchers have observed seizures and abnormally high levels of neurotransmitters after feeding laboratory animals massive doses of aspartame. (Used in normal amounts, however, the sweetener is harmless.) Aspartic Acid is also an ingredient in detergents, fungicides, and germicides.

Avoid if . . .
Because of its many potential effects, Aspartic Acid should be used only by healthy adults, for short periods—a few weeks at a time. If you have an existing medical condition, use only under your doctor's supervision. Children should not be given Aspartic Acid without a doctor's supervision.

Special Cautions
Check with your doctor before taking Aspartic Acid if you have any medical problems.

Possible Drug Interactions
No interactions have been reported.

Special Information if You Are Pregnant or Breast-feeding
Aspartic Acid is not recommended for use by pregnant or breast-feeding women without a doctor's supervision.

Available Preparations and Dosage
Currently, Aspartic Acid is used in high doses. Proponents suggest 2 to 4 grams a day for short periods, under a doctor's supervision.

Overdosage
Toxic levels have not been established, and there is no information on the effects of an overdose.

Bee Pollen

Why People Take It

Pollen extracts have been used for many years to detect allergies, but it is only during the past few years that Bee Pollen has gained popularity as a nutritional supplement.

Promoted as an energy booster and general tonic for better health, vitality, and happiness, it does in fact contain vitamins, minerals, sugar, protein, and fat—but not in exceptional quantities. For instance, claims that it is an outstanding source of protein are, to say the least, exaggerated. Despite its extravagant cost per pound, it's no better than a variety of common sources.

Some athletes take Bee Pollen in the belief that it increases their strength, endurance, energy, and speed. It's said to help the body recover from exercise by returning breathing and heart rate to normal and improving endurance for repeat exertion. It is also promoted as a metabolic booster, to increase the speed at which calories are burned and eliminate excess weight. Unfortunately, scientific tests have failed to detect any improvement in performance due to Bee Pollen.

Reports that Bee Pollen slows the aging process and increases longevity also appear unduly optimistic. The belief is based on the long lives of an isolated clan of mountain people who, when studied closely, didn't appear to consume any Bee Pollen whatsoever.

A variety of other claims seem equally baseless. Bee Pollen has been promoted as a remedy for weakness, anemia, neurasthenia, brain damage, cerebral hemorrhage, indigestion, enteritis, colitis, and constipation, but studies confirming its effectiveness for such problems are conspicuously absent. Likewise, its use as a remedy for allergies seems debatable. Although it's said to reduce production of the histamine involved in allergic reactions, it has in fact *caused* allergic reactions in some individuals.

What, then, is Bee Pollen good for? Studies conducted in Sweden and Japan seem to indicate that it might be of value in treating chronic prostate problems. And an Austrian report claims that it's useful in alleviating the symptoms of radiation sickness in patients treated for cervical cancer. However, all such isolated studies require further confirmation.

What It Is; How It Works

Pollen consists of microspores, the male reproductive elements of seed-bearing plants. Although the "Bee Pollen" label on many commercial supplements implies that it was collected from various plants by honeybees, that may not necessarily be the case. While a trap does exist that brushes off and collects the pollen carried on the back legs of bees as they reenter the hive, there's no way to determine whether a particular pollen grain was collected in this way or not.

Although the constituents of pollen vary greatly, depending on the originating plant species, season of the year, and harvest methods, Bee Pollen typically contains a broad spectrum of nutrients. Promoters say that the vegetable protein in the product includes at least 18 amino acids (and all 8 essential amino acids). The pollen is also said to contain more than a dozen vitamins including B complex, A, C, D, and E; 28 minerals; 11 enzymes and coenzymes; and 11 carbohydrates.

Although this sounds impressive, an ordinary balanced diet provides all these nutrients and more—while sparing you from the insect eggs and droppings, fungi, and bacteria that often contaminate pollen. Remember, too, that while any of the nutrients in these products may indeed have therapeutic value when taken individually in purified form, when mixed together in pollen they have yet to exhibit any clinically proven benefits.

Avoid if . . .
Avoid all bee products if you're allergic to bee stings.

Special Cautions
If you have seasonal allergies, keep in mind that pollen can trigger an allergic reaction whether inhaled or eaten. The possibility of any therapeutic benefit you might receive from pollen could be more than outweighed by the danger of a serious reaction. Especially for people with a heart condition or a serious infection, experiments with pollen are not worth the risk.

Possible Drug Interactions
No information on interactions is available.

Special Information if You Are Pregnant or Breast-feeding
No specific information is available. However, it's wise to check with your doctor before taking any supplement while pregnant or breast-feeding.

Available Preparations and Dosage
Bee Pollen is available in granule form, and in capsules and tablets ranging from 500 to 1,000 milligrams. Manufacturer's dosage recommendations vary. One typical dosage of granules is 32 grams.

Overdosage
No information on overdosage is available.

Bee Propolis

Why People Take It
Therapeutic properties have been ascribed to Bee Propolis since the dawn of medicine, when Hippocrates recorded its effectiveness in healing wounds. The ancient Romans and Egyptians revered the bee, and commonly consumed

Propolis both as a remedy and for its health benefits. Today advocates recommend taking it internally as a health enhancer or applying it externally for skin disorders.

Those who favor the use of Propolis as a dietary supplement call it nature's antibiotic. And, indeed, the substance does exhibit some anti-inflammatory, antibacterial, antiviral, and antifungal effects in lab tests and trials in small animals. Its effectiveness in humans, however, has yet to be verified.

What It Is; How It Works

Bee Propolis starts out as tree resin, the waxy coat that protects new tree growth. Bees harvest the resin and combine it with their own secretions to produce a dark gluelike substance that is used in the building and repair of the hive. Bees coat each cell of the hive with a layer of Propolis to protect the contents against invading microorganisms and other environmental threats to the health of the hive.

Laboratory analysis shows that Propolis is half made up of resins gathered from various trees and other plants, with the rest a mixture of beeswax, oils, and pollen. It contains amino acids, enzymes, vitamins, and minerals. Advocates suggest that it may provide protective effects for humans in much the same way it guards the health of the hive. They report that it shows the ability to prevent the growth of certain microbes in laboratory cultures, including influenza and herpes viruses and some bacteria responsible for upper respiratory infections.

Propolis is also rich in flavonoids (pigments that give color to plants), which are known for their antioxidant effects. Flavonoids were discovered in the middle of the twentieth century, and by later decades researchers had found that they not only play a role in the prevention of cell damage from oxidation, but also tend to promote nutrient absorption, support the immune system, and reduce inflammation.

This array of purported beneficial properties prompts some advocates to suggest that Propolis could prove useful in the treatment of heart disease, high blood pressure, arthritis, and asthma. Some also recommend it for stomach ulcers, burns, acne, herpes, and certain diseases of the eyes, mouth, and throat. At this point, however, its medicinal value must still be considered theoretical.

Avoid if . . .
Do not use Bee Propolis if you have a history of allergic reaction to bee stings or bee products.

Special Cautions
Some people are highly allergic to bee products. Make your first dose of Bee Propolis very small, and be alert for warning signs of an allergy. If a rash or swelling develops, stop using the product. If you feel faint or have difficulty breathing, seek emergency attention immediately.

Possible Drug Interactions
No interactions have been reported. Because Bee Propolis is often used in combination with other herbs and minerals, be sure you know all the ingredients in the preparation.

Special Information if You Are Pregnant or Breast-feeding
No harmful effects are known. However, it's best to check with your doctor before taking any supplement during this critical period.

Available Preparations and Dosage
There are no guidelines for taking Bee Propolis. Manufacturers generally recommend 750 milligrams daily, divided into smaller doses. The supplement can be taken in tablet, capsule, tincture, or lozenge form. Propolis is also available in tinctures, sprays, and ointments for external use.

Overdosage
No information on overdosage is available.

Beta-Glucan

Why People Take It
Beta-Glucan has prompted medical research on several fronts. In Japan and China, doctors have found that Beta-Glucan derived from certain mushrooms can extend the survival of patients with some cancers, while minimizing symptoms caused by the cancer itself or the toxic therapies used to treat the disease. (Indeed, in

Japan two forms of this substance—namely, lentinan and schizophyllan—have been approved for clinical use in the treatment of cancer patients.) However, there is no evidence that Beta-Glucan supplements can *prevent* the development of tumors.

Meanwhile, in 1997, the U.S. Food and Drug Administration singled out Beta-Glucan in the soluble fiber of whole oats as the compound responsible for lowering levels of "bad" LDL cholesterol. (However, even though the FDA acknowledged that Beta-Glucan from other sources—such as Beta-Glucan supplements—might have a similar effect, it said that more evidence was needed before such products could be considered effective.)

In addition, laboratory and animal studies have determined that Beta-Glucan can protect against certain viruses and bacteria. This finding has led Beta-Glucan's more enthusiastic advocates to suggest that the supplement can benefit all people whose immune systems have been compromised—people with HIV/AIDS and those under physical or emotional stress, for example. Many proponents recommend taking daily doses of Beta-Glucan to ward off infection and repair and rejuvenate the skin. However, the supplement's anti-infective properties have not been proven in humans, and little research exists to support immune-boosting claims.

What It Is; How It Works
Beta-Glucan is a polysaccharide (a complex carbohydrate) found in the cell walls of plants, fungi, and certain bacteria. Over-the-counter Beta-Glucan supplements are typically derived from yeast or mushrooms.

Beta-Glucan's effect on the immune system remains to be clarified. However, one prominent theory suggests that it boosts immunity by binding to the body's macrophages, the white blood cells that seek and destroy foreign invaders such as bacteria and viruses. Once this binding occurs, it is thought that the immune system's other weapons—including natural killer cells, neutrophils, and cytokines—will spring into action.

Avoid if . . .

Researchers have yet to uncover any toxic effects. However, if you are allergic to yeast, you might want to approach some Beta-Glucan supplements with caution. Products derived from *Saccharomyces cerevisiae*, also known as baker's yeast, may not be purified enough to prevent a reaction.

Special Cautions

Beta-Glucan derived from *Coriolus versicolor*, a mushroom, has been known to produce the occasional darkening of the fingernails in cancer patients—the only significant side effect to date.

Possible Drug Interactions

No drug interactions are known.

Special Information if You Are Pregnant or Breast-feeding

No information is available on the effect of Beta-Glucan during pregnancy or breast-feeding. Check with your doctor before using it during this critical period.

Available Preparations and Dosage

Beta-Glucan is available in capsule, tablet, powder, and liquid form. (The supplement is also an ingredient in some creams and cosmetics.) Preparations range in strength from 1 to 500 milligrams.

Most clinical trials of Beta-Glucan for cancer therapy involved doses of 3 grams daily.

Overdosage

No information on overdosage is available.

Bifidobacterium Bifidum

Why People Take It

Just mention the word "bacteria" to most people, and they think "disease." But not all bacteria are bad for you. A variety of "good" bacteria are permanent tenants in the human body and help maintain its health. Collectively, these friendly bacteria are known as probiotics (which means "for health").

Bifidobacterium bifidum (B. bifidum), together with other probiotics—including *B. longum, Lactobacillus acidophilus, L. bulgaricus, L. sporogenese,* and *Streptococcus thermophilus*—work together with the body's own defenses to promote good digestive health and increase resistance to infections. There's also at least some evidence to suggest that these beneficial bacteria may normalize hormone levels, reduce cholesterol, and protect against some forms of cancer.

What It Is; How It Works

In the healthy human being, colonies of *B. bifidum* typically inhabit the vagina and the lower part of the small intestine, where they synthesize B vitamins (thiamin, riboflavin, pyridoxine) and vitamin K, decrease the pH— thereby increasing the acidity—of the intestines to levels that discourage harmful bacteria, and produce substances that suppress their growth.

Unfortunately, good bacteria can easily be killed by antibiotics or overrun by harmful bacteria from food and the environment. There is strong evidence that the numbers and efficiency of these bacteria decline as we age. And people eating a poor diet or suffering from diarrhea can loose millions of probiotics. The absence of these bacteria enables harmful germs to grow out of control, causing all sorts of health problems, from yeast infection to constipation.

The good news is that there are a number of ways— from diet to supplements—to ensure that you maintain an optimal level of beneficial bacteria, including *B. bifidum*. In addition to eating a healthful diet (low in refined sugars and high in fresh fruits and vegetables), you may want to increase the amount of yogurt in your diet. Choose nonfat or lowfat yogurt with live, active cultures.

If you're interested in using a supplement, consider one

that combines several types of probiotics (for example, *Lactobacillus* plus *Bifidobacterium*) and read the label to ensure that the manufacturer guarantees potency and stability. Most formulas need to be refrigerated. Your supplement should also contain fructo-oligosaccharides (FOS), a nonnutritive sugar that serves as a source of energy for *B. bifidum*.

Avoid if . . .
B. bifidum appears to be safe for all ages and genders.

Special Cautions
Most experts advise against taking probiotics continuously. Instead, they recommend reserving them for short courses to repopulate the colon with friendly flora after antibiotic therapy, to treat intestinal yeast overgrowth, or to stave off infectious diarrhea when you are traveling in underdeveloped countries.

    B. bifidum has no serious side effects. When you first start taking any probiotics, you may notice an increase in gassiness or bloating (a sign that the good bacteria are fermenting). Don't worry. Within a week or two, your body will adjust to the change.

Possible Drug Interactions
No interactions are known.

Special Information if You Are Pregnant or Breast-feeding
B. bifidum is generally considered safe during pregnancy and breast-feeding. (In breast-fed infants, in fact, *Bifidobacterium* may account for 90 to 100 percent of the total population of friendly bacteria.)

Available Preparations and Dosage

B. bifidum supplements typically come in capsule, liquid, or powder form. "Probiotic" formulations contain from 2 to 12 billion cells per daily dosage. "Multinutrient" formulas usually have a lower cell content: from 250 million to 2 billion cells.

While counts of 300 to 500 million cells have been shown to be clinically effective, some authorities have claimed as many as 1 billion bacteria are necessary for an effective daily dose. A typical regimen might involve 3 capsules daily, half an hour before meals, or 1 tablespoon of liquid half an hour before meals. Because formulations vary, follow the supplier's directions.

Overdosage

Even in large doses, probiotics don't appear to have any harmful effects.

Bioflavonoids

Why People Take Them

Bioflavonoids, a diverse group of plant-based chemical compounds, have been used historically to treat a variety of conditions, including rheumatic fever, polio, miscarriage, excessive bleeding in childbirth or menstruation, rheumatoid arthritis, gum disease, diabetic retinitis, macular degeneration, and cataracts. They were isolated in the 1930s by Dr. Albert Szent-Györgi, the Hungarian scientist who won the Nobel Prize in Medicine for discovering vitamin C. He found that Bioflavonoids increase that vitamin's effectiveness.

Although Bioflavonoids were frequently prescribed by doctors for the next three decades, all Bioflavonoid drug products were pulled off the market by the Food and Drug Administration in 1968, following a finding that they were ineffective for treating any medical conditions in humans. The FDA did nothing to prevent Bioflavonoids from being sold as food supplements, however, and they have continued to be available, usually in combination with vitamin C.

Recently, Bioflavonoids have regained some of their mid-twentieth-century popularity. Clinical research studies in humans have shown that substances contained in Bioflavonoids may be helpful in treating varicose veins and easy bruising, and certain eye conditions as well. A Bioflavonoid substance found in extracts of both grape seed (see separate entry) and pine bark may also play a role in preventing heart disease and stroke.

The association of Bioflavonoids with vitamin C has led to claims that they can help to ward off colds and treat flu. It is also claimed that they play a role, either directly or indirectly through vitamin C, in maintaining the health of the collagen that helps to bind human cells, tissues, and cartilage. Some claim that it may therefore have some effect on the pain, bumps, and bruises commonly caused by athletic injuries. However, there's little scientific evidence to support these claims.

Certain individual Bioflavonoids have commanded a flurry of interest recently. Proponents of green tea as a health remedy claim that the Bioflavonoid polyphenols it contains have anticancer, antioxidant, antibacterial, and antiviral properties. However, these compounds are found not just in green tea, but in all plants, and their beneficial effects in humans remain unproven.

Another Bioflavonoid, catechin, is under study as an allergy remedy. Advocates claim—without convincing evidence—that it also helps to protect the liver from the effects of alcohol and helps cure people with hepatitis B. Similar claims are made for the Bioflavonoid quercetin. This compound is also said to be helpful in combating the effects of bursitis, arthritis, asthma, prostate problems, and tissue trauma. Some think that it may decrease the infectiousness of certain RNA and DNA viruses, such as herpes, polio, and Epstein-Barr. Unfortunately, all these possibilities are far from proven.

What They Are; How They Work

Bioflavonoids can be found in a variety of fruits and vegetables, where they provide much of the pigment that lends the plants their color. They usually accompany vitamin C, and have a positive effect on its absorption and processing. Among the more important Bioflavonoid compounds are hesperidin, nobeletin, rutin, sinensetin, tangeretin, quercetin, catechin, genistein, and citrus Bioflavonoids.

Advocates of Bioflavonoids claim that most of their benefits stem from their ability to increase the strength of the capillaries and to regulate their permeability, an effect first noted by their discoverer, Dr. Szent-Györgi. The effect on capillary permeability is also the source of claims for the usefulness of Bioflavonoids in preventing stroke and eye diseases.

Some researchers believe that Bioflavonoids also have antioxidant properties, mopping up the by-products of metabolism (free radicals) that often receive blame for tissue damage and the aging process. In particular, the purported anticancer effects of green tea and especially grape seed extract are commonly ascribed to their antioxidant action.

Advocates also claim that some Bioflavonoids restrain the activity of certain compounds that cause inflammation in the body, such as the histamines associated with allergy and a compound that causes cataracts. For example, it is this property that is supposedly responsible for quercetin's effectiveness against prostate inflammation.

Bioflavonoids are found in soybeans, citrus fruits, root vegetables such as potatoes and onions, rose hips, black currants, grapes, apricots, strawberries, cherries, plums and prunes, buckwheat, green peppers, tomatoes, and nuts. Conservative nutritionists insist that Americans get enough Bioflavonoids in their everyday diet to meet their needs, and that supplements are unnecessary.

Avoid if . . .
There are no known reasons to avoid *ordinary* amounts of Bioflavonoids.

Special Cautions

Test-tube research indicates that heavy doses of some Bioflavonoids may cause genetic damage in the very young and may be linked with leukemia in infants and children. Most adult leukemia involves a different sort of genetic damage and therefore Bioflavonoids are not associated with its onset. Otherwise, Bioflavonoids have no known toxicity.

Possible Drug Interactions

Bioflavonoids are not known to have any adverse drug interactions.

Special Information if You Are Pregnant or Breast-feeding

Due to their association with genetic damage, megadoses of Bioflavonoids should be strictly avoided during pregnancy.

Available Preparations and Dosage

There is no official recommended dietary allowance for Bioflavonoids. They are often included in vitamin C supplements, which provide many people with their main source of the compounds, and can be found in many multivitamin supplements as well.

When they are taken as supplements apart from vitamin C, a typical dosage is 500 milligrams—including 50 milligrams of rutin and 50 milligrams of hesperidin—taken 1 to 3 times daily. Supplements containing 125 or 250 milligrams of Bioflavonoids are also available, and may be taken on the same schedule.

Overdosage
Bioflavonoids have no known overdose effects.

Bone Meal

Why People Take It
As you might have guessed, Bone Meal is used primarily
as a calcium supplement. (Some makers also advertise
it as a source of magnesium, vitamin D, phosphorus, and
other minerals, and some preparations have other vitamins added.)

Everyone knows that calcium is needed for strong
bones and teeth. But it also aids in the transmission of
nerve impulses, and enables muscles—such as the heart—
to relax and contract. It helps to maintain the body's acid
balance, assists in the clotting process, strengthens cell
membranes, and aids in the passage of nutrients and
other substances in and out of cells.

Depending on their age and gender, people need from
1,000 to 1,300 milligrams of calcium daily—and many
don't get enough. A shortage of calcium can cause muscle
cramps, brittle nails, eczema, aching joints, arthritis,
heart palpitations, and numbness in the arms and legs.
Over the long term, it can lead to internal bleeding, tooth
decay, and the brittle-bone disease osteoporosis.

Given the host of benefits that calcium confers, you'd think that Bone Meal would be highly recommended. Actually, quite the opposite is true. The U.S. Food and Drug Administration and many other authorities strongly warn against the use of Bone Meal. Why? Because in addition to a host of beneficial minerals, it often contains lead.

Lead is especially dangerous for children and pregnant women. Yet an analysis of 70 brands of calcium supplements found that about a quarter of them exceeded the FDA's total allowable lead intake level for children aged 6 and under. Bone Meal supplements were among the highest in lead content.

What It Is; How It Works

Bone Meal is simply animal bones, primarily beef bones, ground to a powder. A number of early health food advocates assumed that Bone Meal would be a superior mineral supplement because animal bones have much the same composition as human bones. However, most research shows that the calcium in Bone Meal is *not* well absorbed, and that a number of other over-the-counter calcium supplements are at least as good or better.

Actually, the best way to increase your calcium intake is to add calcium-rich foods to your diet. Scientists say that the body absorbs minerals obtained from food more effectively than it does minerals in supplement form. The best dietary sources of calcium are dairy foods, because they also contain vitamin D and lactose, which help the body to absorb calcium. Salmon, sardines, and leafy green vegetables are other good sources.

If your diet still leaves you short of calcium and you want to try Bone Meal as a natural supplement, read the label carefully. Some brands advertise that they are safe because they are derived from the bones of specially treated calves raised in a chemical-free environment. Check, too, to see whether the product is imported. Concerns about bovine spongiform encephaly, the "mad cow disease" that contaminated British beef in the 1990s may be relevant here. Also make sure that the Bone Meal is labeled for human consumption, and not for pets or plants.

To check any calcium supplement for proper absorbability, drop a tablet into a container with 2 to 4 ounces of vinegar and stir twice. After 30 minutes, the pill should have completely dissolved or disintegrated into fine particles. If not, change brands.

Avoid if . . .
Anyone with cancer, hyperparathyroidism, sarcoidosis, or a tendency to develop kidney stones should take calcium supplements only under a doctor's supervision.

Special Cautions
The body can generally tolerate up to 2,000 milligrams of calcium daily, although that's more than it needs. Beyond that, calcium can build up in the body in painful deposits. Early warning signs of calcium overload include loss of appetite, constipation, dry mouth or a metallic taste in the mouth, headache, drowsiness, and a feeling of weakness or fatigue.

Possible Drug Interactions

There are no known specific drug interactions with Bone Meal. However, you may need extra magnesium and vitamin D to make optimal use of the calcium in Bone Meal. Remember, too, that calcium supplements should not be taken at the same time as iron supplements. Calcium can interfere with the absorption of iron.

Special Information if You Are Pregnant or Breast-feeding

Due to the possibility of contamination, it's especially important to avoid Bone Meal while you're pregnant or breast-feeding.

Available Preparations and Dosage

For proper absorption, the National Institutes of Health recommend that calcium intake be limited to 500 milligrams per dose, and that doses be taken between meals. A number of manufacturers offer Bone Meal in tablet or powder form, with recommendations of about 5 grams per dose. Check the calcium content; 1,000 milligrams of Bone Meal provides significantly less than 1,000 milligrams of calcium.

Overdosage

A single massive dose of calcium is unlikely to cause serious problems, However, an overdose of the magnesium in Bone Meal may cause diarrhea, and in extreme cases could lead to kidney failure.

Branched-Chain Amino Acids

Why People Take Them

Like all amino acids, the three in the so-called branched-chain group are building blocks of protein. Fitness enthusiasts take them to build muscle. They say they reduce fatigue, permitting longer workouts. They also believe that these compounds minimize the amount of "muscle repair" needed after a strenuous workout. But, while there's some evidence that Branch-Chain Amino Acids may in fact help restore muscle mass after surgery or an injury, their value in bodybuilding has yet to be verified in clinical trials.

What They Are; How They Work

The three Branched-Chain Amino Acids—leucine, isoleucine, and valine—are classified as "essential," because the body is unable to manufacture them and they must be obtained from the diet. Each of these amino acids plays a different role in the body:

Isoleucine serves as raw material for certain chemicals used in the production of energy. It also contributes to the formation of oxygen-carrying hemoglobin and helps regulate the body's blood sugar levels. The estimated safe and adequate daily intake is about 6 milligrams per pound of body weight. Infants require more than three times that amount per pound of body weight; children require twice the adult amount.

Leucine is essential for growth. It boosts the production of growth hormone and lowers elevated blood sugar levels by stimulating insulin secretion. The estimated safe and adequate daily intake is about 9 milligrams per pound of body weight. Infants require almost five times that amount per pound of body weight; children require approximately twice the adult amount.

Valine, along with the other two in the group, is a constituent of most of the body's proteins. The estimated safe and adequate daily intake is about 6 milligrams per pound of body weight. Infants require more than four times that amount per pound of body weight; children require approximately twice the adult amount.

Branched-Chain Amino Acids are plentiful in most meat and dairy products, and most healthy adults get all they need from their diet. A deficiency of protein and amino acids would be signaled by a loss of stamina, lowered resistance to infection, slow healing of wounds, weakness, and depression.

Avoid if . . .

High doses of amino acids lay an extra burden on the liver and kidneys. If you have a problem in either area, don't take this product without your doctor's approval.

Special Cautions

For adults, even large amounts of amino acids are unlikely to cause any side effects. However, some infants are unable to process the Branched-Chain Amino Acids properly and develop a problem called "maple syrup urine disease." The first sign of trouble is an odor of maple syrup from the child's urine. Left untreated, the condition can quickly lead to convulsions, coma, and death. Stringent dietary restrictions are needed to overcome the problem.

Possible Drug Interactions

No drug interactions have been reported.

Special Information if You Are Pregnant or Breast-feeding

Scientists have not studied the effects of Branched-Chain Amino Acid supplements during pregnancy. Since you don't need these supplements to maintain good health, the safest course is to avoid them while pregnant or breast-feeding.

Available Preparations and Dosage

Combinations of the three amino acids are available in tablet form. For muscle building, suppliers typically recommend 3 to 6 tablets, taken before meals and after a workout.

Overdosage

No information on overdosage with Branched-Chain Amino Acids is available. However, excessive leucine can cause low blood sugar and boost the body's ammonia levels.

Brewer's Yeast

Why People Take It

Rich in B vitamins, amino acids, and chromium, Brewer's Yeast has long been recommended for maintaining the body's fitness and resistance. It's used as a remedy for minor infections such as coughs and colds, sore throat, bronchitis, acne, and boils. It's also taken for chronic indigestion and poor appetite.

Because of its high chromium content, some researchers feel it could prove helpful for diabetes, lowering blood sugar levels and reducing the need for insulin and oral diabetes drugs. Some studies indicate that the chromium in Brewer's Yeast can also lower cholesterol levels. And, due to its impact on the immune system and the bacteria that inhabit the intestines, Brewer's Yeast often proves helpful in cases of infectious diarrhea.

What It Is; How It Works

Brewer's Yeast is a powdered preparation of *Saccharomyces cerevisiae*, a type of fungus employed in brewing beer. It has been used since antiquity, in all probability, both for the preparation of alcoholic beverages and as a medication.

Brewer's Yeast grows worldwide and is found extensively in the wild. It is, in fact, an independently living plant, but was not recognized as such until the nineteenth century. Its effectiveness as a health remedy was first confirmed in 1886. Researchers have found that it has antibacterial properties and that it promotes production of certain white blood cells.

Avoid if . . .

People with severely weakened immune systems should avoid unsterilized Brewer's Yeast. Contaminants in the product could cause infection.

Special Cautions

If you are prone to migraine headaches, use Brewer's Yeast with caution; it can trigger migraines in susceptible people.

Large quantities of Brewer's Yeast can cause gas. In some people it prompts allergiclike reactions such as itching, skin eruptions, rashes, and swelling.

Possible Drug Interactions

Brewer's Yeast can trigger an increase in blood pressure if you take it with a drug classified as a monoamine oxidase

(MAO) inhibitor, such as the antidepressants Nardil and Parnate and the Parkinson's disease medication Eldepryl.

Special Information if You Are Pregnant or Breast-feeding

No harmful effects are known. However, it's best to check with your doctor before taking any supplement during this critical period.

Available Preparations and Dosage

Brewer's Yeast is often taken in powder form, but is also available in tablets. Dosage recommendations range from a teaspoonful to 1 to 2 tablespoonfuls daily. Since potency may vary, check the manufacturer's recommendations.

Overdosage

No information on overdosage is available.

Caprylic Acid

Why People Take It

Caprylic Acid supplements are often taken to increase or rebalance the "good" bacteria that live in the intestinal tract, and to fight yeast infections such as *Candida albicans*. However, the effectiveness of Caprylic Acid for these purposes has yet to be established scientifically.

A type of saturated fatty acid, Caprylic Acid is more easily digested and absorbed than some other varieties of fat. As a result, an oil form of Caprylic Acid is sometimes used as a dietary supplement for individuals with disorders that interfere with the absorption of nutrients.

Recent studies suggest that Caprylic Acid may also have beneficial effects on high blood pressure, although scientists are not certain why.

What It Is; How It Works

Caprylic Acid occurs naturally in a number of foods, including butter and coconut oil. It's also one of the fatty acids found in the oil of the saw palmetto berry, which is used as a natural remedy for prostate enlargement.

Caprylic Acid gets its name from goat's milk, which contains it; the word "caprylic" comes from *capparis*, the Latin word for goat. Also known as octanoic acid, it's known to increase the acidity in the bowel—an action that may have suggested its advocates' claims of intestinal benefits.

Caprylic Acid is often added to processed foods such as baked goods, frozen dairy desserts, snack foods, and candy. It's also an ingredient in many soaps, lotions, and other cosmetic products. It softens the skin and has a mild exfoliating effect that promotes the sloughing-off of dead skin cells. It is considered gentle to sensitive skin.

Avoid if . . .

Some experts recommend avoiding Caprylic Acid if you have diabetes or an illness affecting the liver.

Special Cautions

Large doses of Caprylic Acid can cause diarrhea. Supplement suppliers also caution that a few individuals taking Caprylic Acid may experience mild to severe fatigue, headaches, nausea, flulike aches, a generally ill feeling, itching, and hives.

Possible Drug Interactions

If you are taking a drug for high blood pressure, check with your doctor before taking this supplement.

Special Information if You Are Pregnant or Breast-feeding

Researchers have not studied the effects of this supplement during pregnancy. No harmful consequences are known, but during this crucial period it's wise to avoid any supplement that isn't specifically recommended.

Available Preparations and Dosage

Caprylic Acid comes in capsule and tablet form, usually in strengths of 300 to 400 milligrams. Some capsules are coated to prevent release of the ingredients until they've reached the intestinal tract. A number of preparations include a variety of herbs.

The suppliers' dosage recommendations vary. Higher doses are usually recommended if the problem is yeast infection. The supplement is typically taken with meals 2 or 3 times per day.

Overdosage

Excessive doses can cause stomach upset, nausea, and diarrhea. Check with your doctor if you suspect an overdose.

Carnitine

Why People Take It

Carnitine is one of the chemical workhorses of human metabolism. It helps the body transport fatty acids into tiny structures within cells called mitochondria, where the fatty acids are broken down for energy. Carnitine is found in meat and dairy foods, but even vegetarians usually have enough of it, because the human body can manufacture its own supply. That hasn't stopped proponents from touting Carnitine supplements, usually in a form called levocarnitine (or L-carnitine). Another form, called L-acetyl-carnitine, has been investigated for possible use in slowing the progression of Alzheimer's disease.

Carnitine is popular among bodybuilders, who say it boosts stamina and energy while helping weight loss. Advocates claim that it also promotes heart health (particularly for people with congestive heart failure), boosts immunity, and increases sperm quality to combat male infertility. Some of these claims are based on intriguing preliminary research in animals and humans, but Carnitine isn't cheap, and there's still not enough evidence to justify recommendations for supplementation unless you have a medically diagnosed deficiency. However, Carnitine does not appear to be harmful even at relatively high doses.

What It Is; How it Works

Since Carnitine is plentiful in most people's diets and can be built by the body from the amino acids lysine and methionine, deficiencies are rare. When they do occur (usually as a result of liver disease, kidney dialysis, or a genetic disorder), they are treated with a high-grade prescription form of L-carnitine called Carnitor. L-carnitine is also available without prescription in health-food stores and vitamin shops.

None of the benefits claimed for Carnitine have been evaluated by the Food and Drug Administration (FDA) or endorsed by any respected medical authority or organization. The weakest claims are those related to muscle-building and endurance athletics. Carnitine was one of the so-called ergogenic aids whose usefulness was dismissed by the American Dietetic Association in a recent position paper, "Nutrition for Athletic Adults." Although some bodybuilders and other athletes insist these supplements help them, the ADA states that such anecdotal reports are not supported by sufficient scientific evidence from clinical trials, and may arise from nothing more than belief in the product (the "placebo effect").

On the other hand, L-carnitine may have a genuine role to play in the treatment of infertility—at least in cases where either the cause is unknown after a thorough workup, or the cause is known to relate to a man's low sperm count or poor sperm motility (the sperm's ability to move). Seminal fluid has extremely high levels of carnitine, and clinical studies have shown that about 3 grams a day of L-carnitine combined with L-acetyl-carnitine, taken for up to six months, significantly increased sperm count and motility, with some impact on pregnancies achieved.

In people whose hearts have been weakened by an outright Carnitine deficiency, L-carnitine supplements often clear up the problem. Some research suggests that L-carnitine may also help people with congestive heart failure, though Carnitine is not a recognized treatment for this disorder in the United States.

In the form of L-acetyl-carnitine, Carnitine has also shown at least some promise as a treatment for Alzheimer's disease. In a few clinical trials, it seems to have delayed the progression of the disease and temporarily improved mental performance. Doses used were at least 500 milligrams 3 times per day.

Avoid if . . .

While Carnitine may have minimal value for conditions other than deficiency diseases and infertility, there is no known reason, other than pregnancy, for avoiding it.

Special Cautions

If you have reason to suspect a Carnitine deficiency (such as muscle weakness, fatigue, liver disease, or kidney failure), see your doctor for a laboratory test of your Carnitine levels. He or she can prescribe a supplement if necessary. Don't attempt to treat yourself with over-the-counter supplements. Your symptoms could be totally unrelated to Carnitine deficiency.

The L-carnitine supplements prescribed for a deficiency have been known to cause digestive upset (nausea, vomiting, abdominal cramps); large doses may cause diarrhea. The use of L-carnitine has also occasionally been associated with body odor.

Possible Drug Interactions
There are no reported significant drug interactions with L-carnitine.

Special Information if You Are Pregnant or Breast-feeding
Carnitine is considered relatively safe in pregnancy. However, since there's no pressing need for it unless you have a deficiency, it's best to avoid it—and all other unnecessary supplements—when pregnant or breast-feeding.

Available Preparations and Dosage
Nonprescription L-carnitine supplements in tablet or capsule form are available in strengths ranging from 250 to 1,000 milligrams. Supplements of L-acetyl-carnitine are available in 250- to 500-milligram strengths. Pharmaceutical-grade carnitine, a prescription drug, is available in tablet, liquid, or injectable form, for use under a doctor's supervision.

Overdosage
Although large doses may cause unpleasant side effects, no life-threatening overdoses have been reported.

Carnosine

Why People Take It

This amino acid compound is often confused with the sound-alike substance carnitine. And in fact the two do have more in common than their names. Both are favored by bodybuilders, who take them in an effort to boost muscle energy, endurance, and strength, and both are manufactured inside the body from a pair of amino acids. There, however, the similarity ends.

Carnitine is a product of two "essential" amino acids available only in the diet, while Carnosine is built from two "nonessential" amino acids that the body itself can produce. Carnitine seems to act primarily by expediting the conversion of fat into energy. Carnosine, on the other hand, is an antioxidant that appears to have protective effects on muscle tissue and the brain.

Bodybuilders value Carnosine for its ability to retard the formation of lactic acid, the chemical that makes your muscles sore after a hard workout. However, while researchers have verified this effect, they've produced no evidence that Carnosine supplements can improve performance, or can even increase the body's own natural stores.

Carnosine's antioxidant action remains largely unexplored. Preliminary research hints at a variety of exciting possibilities, though none have been confirmed in rigorous clinical trials. Lab experiments show that Carnosine helps protect the brain and may be useful for treating seizures, stroke, and Alzheimer's disease. Proponents claim it could also play a role in controlling blood pressure, regulating the immune system, reducing inflammation, alleviating the complications of diabetes, and combating hardening of the arteries, among other things. In addition, animal studies suggest that Carnosine might be helpful in the treatment of cataracts and skin wounds. All such claims, however, remain unproven and await significant additional research.

What It Is; How It Works

Built from the two nonessential amino acids histidine and alanine, Carnosine is both produced by the body and absorbed from the diet. The best source is meat—just a single serving of beef, pork, or chicken provides 50 to 250 milligrams—but even strict vegetarians have an adequate supply, thanks to the body's own contribution.

Carnosine carries out a variety of duties within the body. In addition to counteracting the effects of lactic acid in the muscles, it appears to contribute to the activation of the muscle fibers. In the brain, it seems to prevent—and even repair—some of the damage done by oxidation, possibly reducing the buildup of waste proteins associated with conditions such as Alzheimer's disease. However, whether supplemental Carnosine has any therapeutic effect remains an open question.

Avoid if . . .

No long-term safety studies have been conducted in humans; therefore, it's not known if certain people should avoid Carnosine. So far, lab tests indicate that it is relatively safe.

Special Cautions

Large doses of some nonessential amino acids can cause nausea, diarrhea, headache, and blood pressure changes. In general, however, even large amounts of amino acids are unlikely to cause any severe reactions, and it's not known whether Carnosine supplements cause any problems at all.

Before taking this supplement, it's wise to check the source. Researchers caution that synthetic Carnosine is sometimes made with toxic materials, including the poisonous compound hydrazine. Buy only pure forms of Carnosine, and check the label to make sure the manufacturer uses formulas based on U.S. patents.

Possible Drug Interactions

It is not known whether Carnosine interacts with medications. If you take any medicine on a regular basis, check with your doctor before taking this supplement.

Special Information if You Are Pregnant or Breast-feeding

The effects of taking extra Carnosine during pregnancy and breast-feeding are unknown. Since it's not needed to maintain short-term health, it's best to avoid using it during this period.

Available Preparations and Dosage

Carnosine is usually found in bodybuilding products or supplements labeled as "performance enhancers." Individual supplements are less common, with dosages varying according to the manufacturer. Some recommend taking Carnosine in several small doses throughout the day to maximize absorption. Follow the directions on the label and check with your doctor if you have any doubts.

Overdosage

No information on overdosage is available.

Cartilage (Shark and Other)

Why People Take It

For centuries, the Chinese have ascribed healthful properties to shark cartilage, taking it in the form of shark fin soup. Today, preparations of cartilage from sharks and cows are sold by numerous companies as unregulated over-the-counter dietary supplements.

Cartilage is promoted for the treatment of joint diseases such as osteoarthritis and other inflammatory conditions such as psoriasis. In addition, cartilage has become a subject of research and controversy for its alleged anticancer properties. Promoters of cartilage products, claiming that "sharks don't get cancer," have taken some intriguing test-tube and animal studies of the substance's effect on cancer cells as a sign that it may help prevent and treat cancer in humans.

Such claims are premature, to say the least. Sharks do get cancer (although less commonly than humans do), and shark or other cartilage has been evaluated as a cancer treatment in very few well-conducted trials in human subjects.

The few clinical trials that have been published in respected medical journals have failed to show proof of any significant benefit. However, shark cartilage has provoked enough legitimate scientific interest to warrant ongoing cancer research. The National Cancer Institute is currently sponsoring a study of liquid shark cartilage extract along with standard chemotherapy and radiation for lung cancer patients. Unlike most previous trials of cartilage products, this one is placebo-controlled (that is, divided into two groups of patients, some of whom take a dummy pill).

What It Is; How it Works

Cartilage is a tough, translucent material found primarily in the joints. In sharks, cartilage forms most of the skeleton. The material is made up of almost half protein, along with carbohydrate (sugar) compounds and calcium. One possible active ingredient in cartilage is chondroitin sulfate, a substance that has been shown in European clinical research to help ease the pain and inflammation of arthritis. (Chondroitin is also sold as a dietary supplement, often in combination with another compound called glucosamine.) Despite promising results with chondroitin, there is little evidence from clinical trials in humans that cartilage itself, in any form, is effective against arthritis, psoriasis, or other inflammatory conditions.

Anticancer hopes for cartilage arose in the 1970s, when several researchers reported that cartilage and other material from sharks might combat cancer in mice. Further studies raised more questions than answers, particularly about the way shark cartilage might do its work. Hope centers on its potential for "antiangiogenesis," the ability to curb the formation of blood vessels that nourish tumors and help them grow. Cartilage, which has no blood supply, was shown in 1983 to contain substances that inhibit the growth of blood vessels in animal tumors.

Some scientists question whether the antiangiogenesis compounds in cartilage can even be absorbed through the digestive system into the human bloodstream at levels high enough to make a difference. Others have suggested that cartilage may deter cancer by inhibiting cell division or boosting the immune system. These claims, too, are based largely on preliminary biochemical research, not trials of actual cartilage products in people with cancer.

Avoid if . . .

Shark cartilage products are generally costly, and there is scant evidence of their health benefits. The American Cancer Society recommends against using them as a treatment for cancer unless you are participating in an independently monitored clinical trial using clinical-quality cartilage. (There are no standards for the purity, potency, or effectiveness of commercially available cartilage supplements.) It would certainly be inadvisable to use cartilage products in place of standard medical treatment for cancer, arthritis, or any other condition.

Special Cautions
Cartilage rarely causes side effects. If any do occur, they are likely to take the form of a bad aftertaste, nausea, indigestion, excessive levels of calcium in the body, fever, and dizziness.

Since the effect of cartilage supplements on young growing bodies hasn't been studied, they are not recommended for children.

Possible Drug Interactions
There are no reports of dangerous interactions between cartilage and any type of drug. Given the high levels of calcium in cartilage, it may be prudent to avoid combining cartilage products and high doses of calcium supplements. As with any new medication, it's wise to alert your doctor when you begin taking cartilage.

Special Information if You Are Pregnant or Breast-feeding
No information is available on the effect of shark cartilage during pregnancy. Since its benefits are questionable, any risk to the developing baby can hardly be justified, and it should be avoided during both pregnancy and breast-feeding.

Available Preparations and Dosage
Shark cartilage is available in dozens of formulations, including capsules, tablets, powders, liquid extracts, enemas, and injectable preparations. Suggested doses are

relatively high; one major manufacturer recommends five to eight 750-milligram caplets a day.

Overdosage

The results of an overdose—if one is possible—are unknown. Given the high doses recommended to achieve even the possibility of a therapeutic effect, overdosage seems an unlikely risk.

CDP-Choline (Cytidine Diphosphate Choline)

Why People Take It

Touted as a stronger type of choline (see separate entry), CDP-Choline is said to offer many of the same benefits. Like choline, it may sharpen the memory and boost learning—two effects that might help stall aging in the brain. Also like choline, it promises to alleviate some movement disorders. It has been tested in people who have trouble carrying out voluntary movements such as walking—people with Parkinson's disease, for example. And it has also been studied as a treatment for involuntary movements such as the continual chewing or writhing motions (called tardive dyskinesia) occasionally triggered by long-term use of antipsychotic drugs.

Unfortunately, results to date have been less than spectacular. A number of studies have detected small improvements when people with Alzheimer's disease, head injury, or tardive dyskinesia were treated with large doses of the substance. Minor benefits have also been observed in studies of people with multi-infarct dementia or stroke—examples of the cerebrovascular diseases that disrupt blood circulation in the brain, robbing it of oxygen. Likewise, some people with Parkinson's disease have enjoyed small improvements in their symptoms when CDP-Choline was added to their regular drug regimen. On balance, though, experts agree that bigger and better studies are needed before CDP-Choline can win a passing grade.

What It Is; How It Works
Routinely present throughout the body, CDP-Choline is a necessary ingredient in the production of compounds known as phospholipids, especially the phospholipid known as phosphatidylcholine. (See separate entry for more on the use of this compound as a dietary supplement.) In turn, phosphatidylcholine and other phospholipids are used to manufacture cell membranes, the barriers protecting the intricate machinery that allows cells to function properly.

Some research suggests that CDP-Choline, like other forms of choline, boosts production of acetylcholine, a chemical messenger (neurotransmitter) that's deficient in the brains of people with Alzheimer's disease. Similarly, CDP-Choline seems to enhance the action of dopamine, the neurotransmitter that's lacking in people with

Parkinson's disease or tardive dyskinesia. Other studies indicate that the drug may somehow protect cell membranes or slow down damage when the brain is deprived of oxygen, as it is in stroke. To some degree, CDP-Choline may also increase the circulation in the brain. At this point, however, all of these possible effects need more research.

Avoid if . . .
Because of its potential impact on neurotransmitters, check with your doctor before using CDP-Choline if you suffer from bipolar disorder or Parkinson's disease. Avoid this product if you're allergic to choline.

Special Cautions
People in research studies have taken as much as 1,000 milligrams of CDP-Choline per day without serious consequences. The most common complaints have been gastrointestinal reactions (nausea, vomiting, diarrhea, stomach pain), dizziness, headache, and fatigue. A small number of people have suffered low blood pressure and changes in heart rate after taking CDP-Choline.

Possible Drug Interactions
CDP-Choline could interfere with the action of drugs that work by blocking the effect of acetylcholine (for example, the antinausea medication scopolamine). Check with your doctor if you're not sure whether you're taking such a drug.

Special Information if You Are Pregnant or Breast-feeding
It is best to avoid any unnecessary medication during pregnancy and breast-feeding. Take only what has been prescribed or recommended by your physician.

Available Preparations and Dosage
Typically, CDP-Choline is sold in capsule form in strengths of 200 to 250 milligrams. Follow directions on the label and check with your doctor if you have any doubts.

Overdosage
No information on overdosage is available.

Chitosan

Why People Take It
Chitosan (pronounced kite-o-san) is used primarily as a dietary supplement to aid in weight-loss programs. Once in the stomach, it is said to attract and bind the fat from food, thereby preventing the body from digesting, absorbing, and storing it.

This product may also help to improve cholesterol profiles by binding with the cholesterol-rich bile produced by the liver, an action that prompts the liver to draw extra cholesterol out of the blood. By reducing levels of "bad" LDL cholesterol and triglycerides, it may help fend off heart disease.

Because it's a type of fiber, it seems to speed elimination of waste, toxins, and undigested fats from the body, thereby relieving constipation and perhaps helping to treat or prevent irritable bowel syndrome. The calcium it contains has also been advocated as a treatment for bowel disease, and even as a cancer preventive.

Chitosan is also purported to reduce blood levels of uric acid, which causes gout. Some say it also promotes healing of ulcers and lesions, has antibacterial properties, fights yeast infections, acts as an antacid, relieves arthritis, and lowers blood pressure, though its practical value for these purposes remains unproven.

What It Is; How It Works

Chitosan is derived from chitin, a substance found in plankton and the shells of crustaceans such as shrimp, crab, and lobster. Like more traditional forms of fiber, it passes through the body without being absorbed. Because it absorbs water, it promotes a full feeling that may lead you to eat less. It also acts as a bulking agent and speeds the transit time of the food we eat; this prevents undigested food and metabolic waste from creating toxic by-products.

Clinical trials have verified Chitosan's weight-loss properties, but only in conjunction with a low-calorie diet that might account for most of the improvement. Its ability to slightly reduce cholesterol levels has also been clinically confirmed.

Avoid if . . .

Do not use Chitosan if you have an allergy or sensitivity to shellfish. Avoid all fiber supplements if you have any type of intestinal obstruction.

Special Cautions

Because Chitosan absorbs water, it's important to drink 6 to 8 glasses per day. Chitosan also tends to bind fat-soluble vitamins, potentially depleting the body's supply; so take a good-quality multivitamin supplement daily.

You might also want to consider supplementing the "friendly" intestinal bacteria *Bifidobacterium bifidum* and Lactobacillus, since Chitosan may reduce the natural population. Animal studies suggest that Chitosan may decrease calcium absorption, so a calcium supplement may be needed as well.

Possible Drug Interactions

Avoid taking medications or nutritional supplements at the same time of day as Chitosan, since the Chitosan can interfere with their absorption and utilization.

Special Information if You Are Pregnant or Breast-feeding

Although no problems have surfaced, it's best for women who are pregnant or breast-feeding to check with their doctor before using any fiber supplement.

Available Preparations and Dosage

This supplement is generally taken in the form of capsules containing 250 to 500 milligrams of Chitosan. Manufacturers typically recommend that you take 2 capsules 10 to

30 minutes before each meal or before eating snacks high in fat.

Overdosage

No information on overdosage is available.

Choline

Why People Take It

Choline is a vitaminlike compound that has recently gained acceptance as an essential nutrient. Although the body can produce a certain amount of Choline on its own, a dietary deficiency can lead to liver and kidney disorders, high blood pressure, and heart disease.

Choline is one of the building blocks of acetylcholine, a key chemical messenger in the nervous system. This fact has led researchers to study it for a wide variety of neurologic disorders, including Huntington's disease, Parkinson's disease, Alzheimer's disease, and tardive dyskinesia.

Choline shows promise as a way to control mood swings and reduce memory loss. Increases in acetylcholine in the brain seem to improve mood, alertness, and mental energy, while low levels are linked to depression and lack of concentration. Many people who use Choline notice an improvement in overall disposition.

Athletes who take Choline-based supplements report greater energy and less fatigue. And researchers have also found that Choline boosts the mood of at least some Alzheimer's patients. (Choline will not, however, cure Alzheimer's, though it might play a role in staving it off.)

Choline is also reported to help prevent or treat liver disorders such as cirrhosis, fatty liver, hepatitis, and damage due to drugs or toxic substances. In addition, it may confer some benefit to those with eczema, kidney and gallbladder disorders, and bipolar disorder. It also appears to have some positive impact on cholesterol levels, although not to the extent of two related compounds, phosphatidylcholine and lecithin.

What It Is; How It Works

Closely related to the B-complex family of vitamins, choline is found in all living cells, where it supports the integrity of cell membranes. In addition to its role in the production of acetylcholine, it aids in the transport of fats into the body's cells. An adequate supply of Choline is essential for proper liver function.

Choline helps the body to form acetylcholine, a chemical used in the transmission of brain impulses between nerves, muscles, and organs, and plays an important role in the workings of the nervous system. It also aids in the metabolism of fats and their movement in and out of cells, and is necessary for proper liver function.

Avoid if . . .

Don't take Choline supplements if you have an ulcer, since they can increase stomach acid. Consult with your doctor before using Choline if you suffer from bipolar disorder or Parkinson's disease.

Special Cautions

Choline is generally safe and nontoxic even at high levels, although megadoses are usually reserved for treating bipolar disorder and other serious psychiatric disorders. High doses (more than 3.5 grams a day) can be counterproductive, actually causing depression in some people, and can lead to a fishy body odor and such side effects as dizziness, nausea, diarrhea, and abdominal cramps. Excess consumption can also overstimulate muscles, leading to tightening in the shoulders and neck and, ultimately, tension headaches.

Possible Drug Interactions

Avoid Choline if you're taking a prescription drug such as scopolamine (an antinausea medication) that works by blocking the effects of acetylcholine.

Special Information if You Are Pregnant or Breast-feeding

For healthy women, Choline supplements are not recommended during pregnancy and breast-feeding.

Available Preparations and Dosage

The new recommended dietary intake (RDI) for Choline ranges from 425 to 550 milligrams per day for adults. Few people suffer an outright deficiency, since Americans' average dietary intake ranges from 500 to 1,000 milligrams daily. However, since many of the foods richest in Choline, such as egg yolks and liver, are also high in cholesterol, intake may be falling among people who watch their cholesterol levels.

Choline is available as tablets, capsules, gel caps, and liquids. The different forms of Choline (bitartrate, chloride, and dihydrogencitrate) vary in potency from 36 to 75 percent Choline. The optimal daily supplemental dose of Choline is often pegged at 250 to 350 milligrams. Aside from eggs and liver, good dietary sources of Choline are wheat germ, lentils, soybeans, cabbage, and cauliflower. Supplements such as lecithin and phosphatidylcholine supply significant amounts of basic Choline. It's also found in brewer's yeast, and is often included in B-complex and multinutrient vitamins or sold in combination with vitamin B_6 or inositol. It should be taken with meals.

Overdosage

A dose of 200 grams or more (one hundred times the typical dose) could prove dangerous. Sustained megadoses of 3,500 milligrams daily or more tend to cause muscle stiffness and digestive upsets.

Chondroitin

Why People Take It

Although many doctors demand further evidence, some osteoarthritis sufferers are convinced that Chondroitin has given them relief. It is said to ease joint pain, reduce inflammation, and even repair the damaged cartilage that cushions the joints.

Because of its beneficial effect on connective tissue, Chondroitin has also been used to treat torn ligaments and tendons. Some advocates even suggest that it can relieve the pain of gout, cure headaches, relieve respiratory ailments and allergies, hasten wound healing, prevent cancer, improve cardiovascular health, and stave off the effects of aging. However, there is no scientific evidence for these additional claims.

What It Is; How It Works

Chondroitin is a complex carbohydrate found in the connective tissue of all mammals. In the resilient cartilage that pads the joints, Chondroitin acts like a magnet, drawing fluid into the tissues. This fluid plays two important roles: it attracts essential nutrients to the area, and it makes the cartilage spongier and better able to absorb shocks. Chondroitin also protects healthy cartilage from premature decline by preventing the production of certain enzymes that weaken connective tissue and defeating other enzymes that stop nutrients from reaching the cartilage.

Many researchers are convinced that Chondroitin strengthens the protein strands that make up connective tissue. There is also some evidence that, because it contains complex sugar molecules called glycosaminoglycans, it not only can reduce inflammation but can actually rebuild cartilage, especially if the tissue has not been totally destroyed. Chondroitin seems to play an active role in reducing the pain that often accompanies osteoarthritis; and, in some cases, it may even eliminate the need for surgery.

Although Chondroitin often works well on its own, it is frequently combined with glucosamine sulfate, a natural sugar involved in the maintenance and production of cartilage. For some people, this combination—or Chondroitin alone—seems to reduce the need for powerful painkillers such as nonsteroidal anti-inflammatories (NSAIDs). However, it doesn't work for everyone, and won't necessarily restore complete mobility.

Avoid if . . .
Suppliers recommend consulting your doctor before giving Chondroitin to children.

Special Cautions
Although Chondroitin contains sugar molecules, it is considered safe for diabetics. Large doses (more than 10 grams a day) may cause nausea.

Possible Drug Interactions

Chondroitin may reduce the tendency of blood to clot. Consult your physician before taking Chondroitin if you are taking an anticoagulant drug such as Coumadin, or if you have a blood-clotting disorder.

Chondroitin may interfere with the action of prescription and nonprescription drugs, herbal preparations, and nutritional supplements. If you are using any of these preparations, talk to your doctor before taking Chondroitin.

Special Information if You Are Pregnant or Breast-feeding

As with any supplement not needed for the relief of an acute medical problem, your safest course is to avoid taking Chondroitin while pregnant or breast-feeding.

Available Preparations and Dosage

Chondroitin sulfate capsules and Chondroitin sulfate/ glucosamine sulfate combination capsules and tablets are found in many health-food stores or can be ordered by mail.

There are no standard dosage guidelines. For osteoarthritis, some advocates recommend 400 milligrams 3 times a day with meals. Others suggest doses ranging from 250 to 1,600 milligrams a day, depending on body weight. Dosage can be adjusted according to your response. If you are overweight or are taking a water pill (diuretic), you may need a larger dose.

Overdosage

No information on overdosage is available.

Chromium Picolinate

Why People Take It

Chromium has a single major role to play in maintaining health: it improves the effectiveness of insulin, enhancing its ability to move blood sugar into the cells, where it's converted to energy. Some researchers believe that because of poor eating habits, overprocessing of foods, and certain farming practices, some Americans have developed a chromium deficiency, and that this has contributed to an increase in adult-onset diabetes. Since the body is slow to absorb ordinary chromium, a more easily used form, Chromium Picolinate, was developed in the lab as a dietary supplement.

Although there's little question that Chromium Picolinate improves the activity of insulin in people with low chromium levels, its role in the treatment of diabetes remains controversial. Several studies have found that Chromium Picolinate can reduce a diabetic's need for medication, but other research has failed to confirm this. As a result, the official position of the American Diabetes Association is that currently there is insufficient evidence to indicate that Chromium Picolinate supplementation stabilizes blood sugar levels in diabetics.

Chromium Picolinate also tends to reduce cholesterol levels, and scientists think it may be a factor in lowering blood pressure in some people. Preliminary studies show that it might also be helpful in preventing bone loss in postmenopausal women.

Because chromium improves the body's ability to burn blood sugar, Chromium Picolinate has also been touted as an energy-booster, and some manufacturers claim that it can burn body fat for weight loss, build muscle mass, and reverse some effects of aging. All such claims, however, have yet to be confirmed by clinical research.

What It Is; How It Works

Chromium is classified as an "essential" nutrient, since it can be obtained only through dietary intake. Good sources include brewer's yeast, wheat germ, beer, American cheese, whole grains, potatoes, apples, meats, and eggs. Thanks to its alliance with insulin, it is sometimes referred to as "glucose tolerance factor." Without it, glucose tolerance becomes unbalanced and blood sugar levels tend to rise, just as they do in diabetes.

The picolinate added to chromium supplements is an amino acid derivative called a "chelator." Chelation of a substance encourages its absorption by the cells. In this case, the chemical binding of chromium and picolinate acts to help insulin enter cells more easily and improves glucose delivery. It is this effect that prompted claims for Chromium Picolinate as a remedy for diabetes. However, most diabetics appear to have an adequate supply of chromium, so it seems unlikely that the supplement will prove to be a universal cure.

Chromium Picolinate may ultimately be found to pose

some long-term risks, as well. Recent studies show that large doses of Chromium Picolinate cause DNA damage in lab animals, possibly increasing the risk of cancer. Workers exposed to chromium have developed skin, liver, and kidney problems, and in some cases, lung cancer. And, while chromium by itself has a low absorption rate, its ready availability in the form of Chromium Picolinate may allow it to accumulate in body tissue and organs, especially the liver. Because so many of its long-term effects have yet to be studied, you might want to check with your doctor before taking the supplement, especially if you are diabetic.

Avoid if . . .
Large doses of Chromium Picolinate have occasionally caused kidney or liver problems. Avoid this supplement if you have kidney or liver disease.

Special Cautions
Although Chromium Picolinate may help keep some cases of diabetes under control, it's no substitute for regular medical treatment. If you have diabetes, continue to follow the plan your doctor recommends, while carefully monitoring your blood sugar.

Possible Drug Interactions
In some diabetics who are chromium deficient, taking Chromium Picolinate can cause a change in insulin requirements. If you feel light-headed after taking Chromium Picolinate, check your blood sugar and adjust your insulin according to your doctor's instructions.

Special Information if You Are Pregnant or Breast-feeding
Women who are pregnant or breast-feeding should not take Chromium Picolinate.

Available Preparations and Dosage
Chromium Picolinate is available in capsule form in strengths ranging from 200 to 1,000 micrograms. While there is no recommended dietary allowance (RDA) for Chromium Picolinate, the estimated safe and adequate daily intake of *chromium* is 50 micrograms to 200 micrograms for adults and children 7 and older. Clinical trials of Chromium Picolinate have used doses of 200 to 1,000 micrograms daily.

Overdosage
Sustained doses of more than 1,000 micrograms daily have, in rare cases, produced kidney and liver problems.

Coenzyme Q10

Why People Take It
For some people suffering from congestive heart failure, irregular heartbeat, or angina, Coenzyme Q10 holds the promise of reduced symptoms and better cardiac function. Some doctors also recommend it after heart surgery

to speed recovery with a minimum of permanent damage. As is true of all other heart medications, however, Coenzyme Q10 is not a cure.

Some advocates contend that Coenzyme Q10 can stave off hardening of the arteries by discouraging the buildup of plaque on artery walls. Others suggest that it can boost the immune system, helping to prevent the spread of cancer. It has also been recommended for a host of additional disorders ranging from high blood pressure, diabetes, allergies, and fatigue to Alzheimer's disease, Bell's palsy, Huntington's disease, Ménière's disease, muscular dystrophy, and deterioration of the retina. However, its effectiveness for all such conditions has yet to be scientifically verified.

What It Is; How It Works

Found in every cell in the body, Coenzyme Q10 plays a vital role in the production of energy, triggering the conversion of nutrients into a "fuel" for the cells to burn. This substance, called adenosine triphosphate (ATP), can't be stored in quantities sufficient to sustain optimum bodily functions for more than a few minutes. Stores must be continually renewed, making an ample supply of Coenzyme Q10 mandatory.

Adequate levels of the enzyme are particularly crucial for the heart because it is constantly in motion, burning twice as much energy as the other organs. If supplies of the enzyme decline, the action of the heart muscle will tend to weaken, reducing the amount of fresh blood the heart can pump out to the body. It is for this reason that some researchers regard a deficiency of the enzyme as an aggravating factor in conditions such as congestive heart failure.

Good dietary sources of Coenzyme Q10 include beef, pork, and lamb; certain types of fish and shellfish; vegetables such as broccoli and spinach; and vegetable oils. If you have a heart condition, however, you may want to consider a commercial supplement.

Avoid if . . .
No known medical condition precludes the use of Coenzyme Q10.

Special Cautions
By itself, Coenzyme Q10 is not a sufficient treatment for any type of heart disease. It is generally employed as a supplement, rather than a replacement, for standard medical therapy. Do not attempt to substitute it for any of your regular prescriptions.

Possible Drug Interactions
No interactions have been reported.

Special Information if You Are Pregnant or Breast-feeding
Do not use Coenzyme Q10 while pregnant or breast-feeding.

Available Preparations and Dosage
Coenzyme Q10 is available in capsule, tablet, gel cap, and chewable form. To improve its absorption, take it with some type of oil (olive oil is recommended) or fat (peanut butter, for example). It is also best to take your dose with meals.

Advocates of Coenzyme Q10 recommend doses ranging from 30 to 400 milligrams daily, generally reserving the higher dose for more severe problems. Large daily doses are typically divided into 2 or 3 smaller doses (for example, one 60 milligram tablet taken 2 times a day instead of a single 120 milligram tablet taken once).

If you are taking the enzyme for a heart condition, it may be 2 to 8 weeks before you notice any benefit, and you will need to continue taking the product to maintain any improvement.

Store in a dry and cool place, away from light. Do not allow to freeze.

Overdosage

Since Coenzyme Q10 is not toxic, experts say you may take large amounts without danger.

Colloidal Silver

Why People Take It

This old-fashioned antiseptic, also known as silver protein, is currently enjoying renewed popularity as an over-the-counter antimicrobial agent and immunity booster. Advocates tout it for a remarkable variety of illnesses.

These include serious ailments such as arthritis, cancer, cholera, diabetes, HIV infection, leprosy, malaria, septicemia (commonly known as blood poisoning), tuberculosis, and ulcers. Other, if less dramatic, conditions supposedly improved by Colloidal Silver include acne, athlete's foot, eczema, herpes infections, prostate problems, rectal itching, runny nose, and yeast infections.

If you think a drug with this many uses seems too good to be true, you're not alone. In September 1999, the U.S. Food and Drug Administration (FDA) banned the use of Colloidal Silver and other silver-based compounds in any nonprescription drug, whether for internal or external use. The reason: Nobody has gathered sufficient scientific evidence to show that any of the claims are true or that people can use colloidal silver on a regular basis without harming themselves.

Nevertheless, a regulatory loophole still allows Colloidal Silver to be sold as a dietary supplement, provided that it meets certain requirements and is labeled properly. For example, to qualify as a dietary supplement, these products must be taken by mouth; something spread on the skin would not be eligible. The label must also carry the following wording: "This statement has not been evaluated by the Food and Drug Administration. This product is not intended to diagnose, treat, cure, or prevent any disease."

Despite these roadblocks, the Internet hosts a number of companies that are attempting to turn silver into gold by promoting Colloidal Silver and its alleged benefits, or by selling special equipment for people who want to make their own Colloidal Silver. Remember, though, that there is currently no proof that this substance will help you in any way—or that it will not hurt you.

What It Is; How It Works
Silver does have the ability to kill germs. Scientists believe that this happens, at least in part, when silver molecules bearing an electric charge attach to a portion of the offending bug and destroy its protective cell membrane.

In Colloidal Silver, tiny particles of silver are evenly dispersed throughout a liquid or solid medium known as the vehicle. (Think of the vehicle as an inactive substance that carries the active ingredient to the site of the problem.) Today's Colloidal Silver products are very dilute, containing minute specks of silver suspended in a vehicle from which they will not readily settle out.

Far more concentrated Colloidal Silver products were used as antiseptics in the first half of the twentieth century before antibiotics were widely available. These would customarily be applied to wounds or to the mucus membranes of the eyes, nose, throat, genitourinary tract, and rectum when patients had an infection, inflammation, or irritation. For example, Colloidal Silver preparations were used to treat inflammation of the urethra caused by gonorrhea. Some people who frequently used these products developed a side effect known as argyria: the skin or mucus membranes took on a permanent blue-gray discoloration, the result of silver deposits in the affected areas.

Today, the use of silver-based drugs is fairly limited. Silver nitrate solution is used in the treatment of stubborn wounds and foot conditions such as plantar warts. In these cases, silver is valued not only for its germicidal properties but for its ability to destroy unnecessary tissue when used in concentrations of 10 percent and higher. A 1 percent solution of silver nitrate is used for newborns to prevent gonorrheal infections of the eyes. Silver sulfadiazine is applied to serious burns in an effort to prevent deadly infections from spreading into the body.

Avoid if . . .

You have ever had an allergic reaction to a silver-based drug.

Special Cautions

Overall, silver does not appear to be toxic when low doses are swallowed or applied to the skin. (Never inject colloidal silver.) The primary concern is argyria, which can occur after prolonged use. While it is not known exactly how much silver can discolor the skin, it has been estimated that argyria can be triggered by taking 25 to 30 grams or more over a 6-month period or by taking a single dose of 3.8 grams. Irritation of the skin or mucus membranes is also possible. Because these agents are being used in ways that have not been studied to any great extent, they might cause adverse effects that have not yet been reported.

Possible Drug Interactions

Colloidal Silver's interaction potential has not been studied.

Special Information if You Are Pregnant or Breast-feeding

It's best to avoid any unnecessary medication during pregnancy and breast-feeding. Take only what has been prescribed or recommended by your physician.

Available Preparations and Dosage

Colloidal Silver is commonly sold as a liquid to be taken by mouth. Strengths and dosages vary. For example, you may find Colloidal Silver in strengths of 10, 20, 30, or 50 parts per million. You may also find products made specifically for use on the skin or note directions suggesting application of an oral product to the skin. Don't confuse such products with approved prescription medications such as Silvaderie Cream, a preparation of silver sulfadiazine used to treat burns.

Overdosage

Swallowing 10 grams of silver or more in a single dose can prove fatal. If you suspect an overdose, seek emergency aid immediately.

Colostrum

Why People Take It

The very first food an infant receives from its mother, Colostrum is rich in a host of life-sustaining compounds such as proteins, vitamins, minerals, amino acids, antibodies, and growth factors. Nature provides this potent mixture to nourish and protect the health of all newborns, human and animal alike. Commercial Colostrum

preparations are promoted primarily as immune enhancers. But Colostrum's array of healthy properties
have inspired marketers to make a variety of other claims
for it—most without scientific basis. Assertions that it
can cure diseases such as cancer, heart disease, multiple
sclerosis, colds, flu, allergies, and arthritis have yet to be
verified by any sort of clinical study.

Human Colostrum is not available for sale, but bovine
(cow) Colostrum is produced and packaged as an over-
the-counter food supplement. Bovine colostrum is an
effective treatment for diarrhea in children who have
been infected with *E. coli* bacteria or rotavirus, with
no apparent side effects. It may also prevent and repair
damage to the stomach lining caused by nonsteroidal
anti-inflammatory drugs (NSAIDs) such as ibuprofen
(Motrin, Advil) and naproxen (Naprosyn). This protective property leads researchers to believe that it could
also be used to treat other gastrointestinal disorders such
as ulcerative colitis and inflammatory bowel disease. In
addition, a recent laboratory study showed that bovine
Colostrum can block *H. pylori*, the bacteria associated
with peptic ulcers.

Some preliminary studies suggest that a component of
Colostrum could also improve cognitive functioning in
people with Alzheimer's disease. But more studies are
needed to confirm this possibility.

What It Is; How It Works

Colostrum is a fluid produced as the primary food source
from a mother's breasts during the first few days after a
baby's birth. The first food introduced to a newborn's
sensitive digestive system, it is sometimes referred to as

foremilk because it precedes the production of breast milk and contains more proteins and antibodies than the regular breast milk that follows. Its rich assortment of nutrients, immune agents, and growth factors offer antiviral and antibiotic properties designed to ensure the survival and health of newborns.

The bovine Colostrum harvested from dairy cows is intended for their own newborn calves. Manufacturers dry and process it into a powdered form. Producers of bovine Colostrum suggest that, just as cow's milk has benefited humans for centuries, it's reasonable to expect that the benefits of bovine Colostrum are transferable as well, and that the product can be well tolerated as a food supplement.

Advocates of Colostrum supplementation base their recommendations on its hoped-for immune-boosting properties. They reason that as we age our bodies gradually produce a diminishing amount of immune and growth factors, and that this results in the decline in the body's ability to repair damaged tissues, fight off disease, and counter the destructive effects of environmental toxins. Since bovine Colostrum is so rich in immunoglobulins, antibodies, and other immune and growth factors, they believe it can confer on adults the same protective effects it bestows on newborns. In addition, they suggest since Colostrum is a balanced, whole food, and not an isolated nutrient that may have unwanted consequences, it may provide health benefits with a minimum of side effects.

While this rationale may sound convincing, actual health benefits (other than those affecting the digestive tract) still need confirmation with human trials. To date, much of the research has been restricted to animals.

Avoid if . . .
There have been no reports of allergic reactions to bovine Colostrum. Still, if you have a dairy allergy or lactose intolerance, use this product with care.

Special Cautions
Colostrum is generally free of side effects.

Possible Drug Interactions
No interactions have been reported. However, Colostrum
products are often combined with other ingredients. Read
the label to make sure you know what you're taking.

Special Information if You Are Pregnant or Breast-feeding
Because commercial Colostrum is not from human
sources, it's best to check with your doctor before taking
one of these products while pregnant or breast-feeding.

Available Preparations and Dosage
Colostrum is available in capsule, tablet, and powder
form in strengths of 500 to 1,000 milligrams. Suppliers
generally recommend dosages of between 500 and 2,000
milligrams per day, the larger amount taken in divided
doses. Colostrum can be taken with or without food.

Overdosage
Colostrum has no known overdose effects.

Conjugated Linoleic Acid

Why People Take It

Conjugated Linoleic Acid (CLA) has been studied for almost two decades. The results have been encouraging in animals, but researchers have only begun to examine what CLA does in humans. Animal research suggests that this fatty acid boosts the immune system and acts as an antioxidant, helping to rid the system of unstable molecules that cause cellular damage. Researchers also note that CLA decreases LDL cholesterol, increases the amount of vitamin A stored in the liver, and seems to prevent diabetes.

Those who swear by CLA, however, are most likely to laud its apparent ability to change the way the body processes food—specifically fat. They believe that CLA acts as a "fat-burner," encouraging the breakdown of fatty acids and leaving less to accumulate as unwanted pounds.

Although several medical uses of CLA are currently under investigation, it is important to note that the U.S. Food and Drug Administration has not yet endorsed the use of CLA for any disease, condition, or purpose.

What It Is; How It Works

Linoleic Acid is a polyunsaturated fatty acid. Polyunsaturated fats have several open chemical links that allow them easily to react with other chemicals and produce energy. (Saturated fats have all their links occupied by hydrogen atoms and aren't as easy to burn.) CLA's purported tendency to provide extra energy while encouraging the burning of fat is the reason it appeals to bodybuilders.

However, extra linoleic acid is hard to come by naturally. It's one of three "essential fatty acids" that the body can't manufacture and that therefore must be obtained from the diet. The foods that contain it—particularly beef and dairy products—are also high in undesirable saturated fats. Hence, the only way to get plenty of Linoleic Acid "uncontaminated" by other fats is to take CLA.

Avoid if . . .

Check with your physician before using Conjugated Linoleic Acid. Advocates warn that CLA increases the activity of a substance called tyrosine kinase C, which helps cancer cells make energy. They recommend that people with cancer use CLA only if they also take a high dose of a substance called soy genistein extract, which is said to counteract this effect.

Special Cautions

Extensive animal research has uncovered no side effects at doses equivalent to 2 to 3 grams of CLA a day.

Possible Drug Interactions

No interactions are known.

Special Information if You Are Pregnant or Breast-feeding
Use of CLA during pregnancy has not been studied, so its safety remains unverified. Like most supplements, it's best avoided during pregnancy unless absolutely necessary.

Available Preparations and Dosage
CLA is available in 1,000-milligram gel caps. A typical regimen is 2 capsules 3 times a day either before or with meals. (Four capsules yield about the same amount of linoleic acid that you would get if you ate 6 pounds of beef or 50 slices of American cheese or a gallon of ice cream.)

Overdosage
No information on overdosage is available.

Creatine

Why People Take It
This popular amino acid compound is used by many athletes and bodybuilders to expand muscle mass, increase short-term muscle strength, and produce quick bursts of energy.

What It Is; How It Works

Creatine (methyl guanidine–acetic acid) is made up of three amino acids: arginine, glycine, and methionine. It is manufactured in the liver, and it can also be found in milk, red meat, and some fish. At any given time, an average 160-pound person has about 120 grams of this compound stored in his or her muscles.

Creatine supplements are thought to provide additional energy for the muscles by bonding with phosphorous stores in muscle tissue to produce creatine phosphate. This substance reacts, in turn, with adenosine diphosphate to create adenosine triphosphate, the chemical that fuels our muscular activity.

In addition, research indicates that Creatine pulls water from the body into the muscles, making them appear larger. Because of this, it's still unclear whether Creatine truly increases muscle fiber or simply inflates the muscles with water. If it's the latter, your muscles are likely to shrink back to normal shortly after you stop taking Creatine.

Some studies suggest that Creatine also acts as a buffer against the lactic acid that builds up in muscles during exercise and eventually causes an intense burning feeling. Others report that it throws the body into an anabolic state that promotes protein synthesis, thereby fostering muscle gain. One study found that Creatine may be beneficial for elderly persons suffering from loss of muscle strength and for those with muscle-wasting diseases such as muscular dystrophy.

Avoid if . . .

Do not use Creatine if you have kidney problems, since it can stress the kidneys. It's best to avoid Creatine, too, if you are trying to lose weight. Because it encourages water retention, people taking it usually put on extra pounds, which is why the supplement is favored more by bodybuilders and football players than, for example, marathon runners.

Special Cautions

Follow the manufacturer's directions closely. Taking more than the recommended amount of Creatine can cause stomach upset and diarrhea. Also, be sure to drink 8 to 12 glasses of water per day while taking Creatine. Because Creatine sequesters water in the muscles, extra fluid intake is needed to prevent dehydration and cramping.

Possible Drug Interactions

There are no reports of interactions with drugs. However, advocates say that Creatine can enhance the effects of other bodybuilding supplements such as whey and glutamine. (See individual entries.)

Special Information if You Are Pregnant or Breast-feeding

There is no information on the effect of Creatine supplementation during pregnancy and breast-feeding. Your safest course is to check with your doctor before taking any supplement during this period.

Available Preparations and Dosage

Creatine is available in powder and liquid formulations. Most manufacturers recommend loading up on the substance with doses totaling 25 grams a day during the first week, then maintaining muscle mass with doses of up to 5 grams a day thereafter. The long-term effects of such doses are unknown; the typical dietary intake is about 2 grams daily.

Overdosage

No information on overdosage is available.

Cysteine

Why People Take It

This nonessential amino acid ("nonessential" because the body can manufacture its own supply if there's none in the diet) helps to maintain and preserve the body's cells. It is a key ingredient of glutathione, an antioxidant that protects cells from damage caused by alcohol, cigarette smoke, pollution, copper, and heavy toxic metals. (See separate entry.) Proponents claim that it staves off hangovers and may even have a protective effect against X rays and nuclear radiation. Recently, some advocates have recommended it for the treatment of arthritis.

Some studies have shown that it strengthens the lining of the stomach and intestines, which might diminish damage caused by aspirin and similar drugs, and which could make it useful in the treatment of gastritis. It also appears to moderate the effects of excess insulin, making it a potential aid in the management of low blood sugar (hypoglycemia). Because hair contains a significant amount of Cysteine, the supplement has also been promoted as a remedy for baldness.

Cysteine also seems to play a role in the proper function of the immune system. Several studies have shown that blood levels of Cysteine and glutathione are low in people infected with HIV.

What It Is; How It Works

Cysteine itself is rarely used as a dietary supplement. Instead, it is usually taken in an altered form called N-acetylcysteine (NAC). NAC helps to break down mucus and has been found useful for people with bronchitis, emphysema, tuberculosis, and chronic obstructive pulmonary disease.

Like Cysteine, NAC helps the body synthesize the antioxidant glutathione, which helps to clear damaging compounds from the liver. In animal studies, it has been found effective against a variety of toxins in the liver. In fact, in emergency rooms NAC is used as an antidote for liver-damaging overdoses of acetaminophen.

Our bodies can build Cysteine from the related antioxidant amino acid methionine. In turn, Cysteine is used to produce taurine, an amino acid that plays an important role in the regulation of the nervous system. Good dietary sources of Cysteine include high-protein food, particularly eggs.

Avoid if . . .
There are no known reasons to avoid normal doses of Cysteine.

Special Cautions
Cysteine is not entirely without risk. Studies involving rats found that extremely large amounts may be toxic to nerve cells. One small study of NAC found that daily amounts of 1.2 grams or more could lead to oxidative damage. Side effects of NAC reported during one clinical trial included nausea, vomiting, headache, dry mouth, dizziness, and abdominal pain.

Possible Drug Interactions
Check with your doctor before taking Cysteine or NAC if you are taking any prescription or over-the-counter medication.

Special Information if You Are Pregnant or Breast-feeding
No specific information is available. However, it's wise to check with your doctor before taking any supplement while pregnant or breast-feeding.

Available Preparations and Dosage
Outright deficiencies of Cysteine are rare, and no recommended dietary allowance exists. For Cysteine itself, proponents often suggest a dosage of 200 milligrams 2 to 4 times daily. For NAC, dosage suggestions range from 250 to 1,500 milligrams daily.

Supplementary Cysteine and NAC are available in capsule, powder, and tablet form. Follow the manufacturer's directions; avoid high doses.

Overdosage

No specific information on overdosage in humans is available.

Desiccated Liver

Why People Take It

Desiccated (dehydrated) liver is a rich source of supplemental protein, B vitamins, and iron. It's also high in vitamins A, C, and D, as well as choline and inositol (see separate entries).

All of these ingredients make essential contributions to our health. Iron is vital for the formation of oxygen-carrying red blood cells, helps the muscles store oxygen, and promotes production of the cellular "fuel" ATP (adenosine triphosphate). B vitamins play a central role in the processing of nutrients and the production of energy. Vitamins A, C, and D respectively maintain the health of the eyes, connective tissues, and bones; choline and inositol aid in the efficient processing of fats.

Small wonder, then, that for half a century body-builders turned to desiccated liver in an effort to add weight and improve muscle tone and endurance. Only in recent years has it been supplanted by other, more sophisticated substances. (Several manufacturers have now discontinued their desiccated liver products.) Still, advisors on nutrition for bodybuilders continue to rate desiccated liver as a good source of protein and vitamins.

Since desiccated liver is a natural product, it hasn't been subjected to the elaborate clinical trials conducted for drugs, and most claims for it are based on the effects of the nutrients it contains. For instance, statements that it aids in recovery from liver disease are based on the beneficial effects that protein, vitamins, and minerals are known to have on the human liver. Likewise, desiccated liver's reputation as a superior source of iron is based on the generally accepted notion that organic iron from animal sources is more readily absorbed than either iron from plants or inorganic mineral iron.

What It Is; How It Works

Desiccated liver is simply beef liver with the water, much of the fat, and the tough connective tissue removed. (Note, however, that it remains high in calories and cholesterol.) Marketers claim that the desiccation process, which requires a relatively low temperature, leaves the nutrients mostly intact, as compared to cooked liver.

Virtually all the desiccated liver on the U.S. market is beef liver, although "swine liver" is sold in Europe. If you've been avoiding beef due to the risk of "mad cow disease" (the viral illness bovine spongiform encephalopathy, detected several years ago in British cattle), you'll probably want to avoid desiccated liver as well. Many of these products are said to be made from high-quality Argentine beef, and are therefore supposedly free of both viral contamination and the growth hormones and antibiotics used on U.S. cattle. Remember, however, that dietary supplements are largely unregulated, so purity cannot be assured. Buy only from a trusted source, look for a disclaimer that health claims have not been evaluated by the Food and Drug Administration, and avoid products with "secret ingredients" such as "antistress factors."

Avoid if . . .
If you have high cholesterol or have been advised to avoid organ meats, check with your doctor before starting a diet regimen that includes desiccated liver.

Special Cautions
No side effects have been reported.

Possible Drug Interactions
There are no known drug interactions.

Special Information if You Are Pregnant or Breast-feeding
No harmful effects are known, and a pure liver supplement could, in fact, be beneficial. Still, it's best to check with your doctor before taking any supplements while pregnant or breast-feeding.

Available Preparations and Dosage
Desiccated liver is usually advertised as being four times as concentrated as regular liver. It's available in tablet, capsule, and powder form. The powder is sold at retail in

containers as large as 10 pounds. The usual capsule size is about 680 milligrams. Some sources advise taking more than a dozen desiccated liver tablets daily.

You'll also find desiccated liver in a variety of combination products. For example, it's frequently combined with other natural substances such as brewer's yeast, and enriched with other vitamins and minerals.

Overdosage
There are no known effects of overdosage. If you experience any adverse effects, check the label for other ingredients.

DHEA (Dehydroepiandrosterone)

Why People Take It
Whether or not DHEA should be taken at all as an unregulated over-the-counter supplement is a controversial issue. There is evidence that DHEA can improve feelings of well-being and increase sexual satisfaction—but only in people whose adrenal glands are functioning poorly. There are also preliminary results indicating that it may have a beneficial effect on some people with major depression.

Much of the controversy arises because DHEA is being

promoted as a cure for many other ailments and has taken on the reputation of an antiaging remedy—a kind of modern-day fountain of youth. Advocates claim that it can help you lose weight; boost your sex drive and immune system; enhance your mood, memory, and energy; and reverse the aging process. Some proponents even suggest using it as an adjunct to conventional cancer therapy. And a number of antiaging clinics recommend taking it as early as your forties or fifties to fight off old age and remain biologically young. Athletes take it in large doses to enhance their performance. However, much of the research behind these claims was done on laboratory animals, and experts caution that the results of such studies are often inconclusive and cannot necessarily be applied to humans. The long-term effects of supplementation are not known, and since DHEA is a powerful hormone, it should be used with great caution and only with your doctor's advice.

What It Is; How It Works

DHEA is a steroid hormone produced primarily by the adrenal glands. It is the most abundant hormone in the body, with the highest concentrations found in the brain. The only known function of DHEA is as a precursor hormone—which means that it is a source material that the body converts into other hormones, such as estrogen and testosterone. It peaks in production by the age of 25 and gradually declines until, by age 70, levels may be more than 80 percent below their earlier highs.

Low DHEA levels have been associated with certain diseases, such as Alzheimer's, cancer, diabetes, multiple sclerosis, lupus, and other immune-function disorders. For this reason, researchers have been tempted to speculate that supplementation with a synthetic form of DHEA could reverse these diseases, much as hormone replacement therapy reduces some of the symptoms of menopause by returning the hormone balance to a premenopausal state. However, it has not yet been proven that either the diseases or the aging process itself are a result of lowered levels of DHEA, and it is not yet clear whether using DHEA is helpful or, in the long run, harmful.

Despite all this, there are physicians who recommend use of this hormone to treat a variety of ailments or combat the effects of aging. If you decide to try DHEA, find a qualified physician to plan and monitor your course of treatment.

Avoid if . . .
You have breast, cervical, uterine, or ovarian cancers, or prostate cancer, or if you have a family history of one of these cancers, since they are hormone related.

Special Cautions
DHEA has been known to cause acne, facial hair growth, and deepening of the voice in some women, and there are reports of breast enlargement in men taking high doses, probably because it triggers hormone production.

Possible Drug Interactions
Check with your doctor about medications you are taking that may be affected by DHEA.

Special Information if You Are Pregnant or Breast-feeding
Because of its hormonal effects, DHEA should not be used during pregnancy or while breast-feeding.

Available Preparations and Dosage
DHEA is available in capsule, tablet, cream, and spray form in strengths ranging from 5 to 200 milligrams.

The dosage should be set by your physician following a blood test or saliva test to determine if your current DHEA level is low, and whether that level is likely to represent a deficiency in you. Based on the results, you may be given 5 to 30 milligrams per day. Your doctor will monitor the level of DHEA in your blood and may adjust the dose as needed.

Overdosage
No information on overdosage is available.

Digestive Enzymes

Why People Take Them
Enzyme supplements have been promoted for an astonishing array of maladies. From acne to AIDS and sciatica to shingles, advocates say Digestive Enzymes are just what's needed to relieve the problem. According to

enthusiasts, even multiple sclerosis, cancer, and aging can be helped by regular enzyme supplementation.

Is there any truth to these claims? The good news is that the supplements can indeed be helpful—if you have one of the rare conditions that cause enzyme deficiency. (Cystic fibrosis, Gaucher's disease, and celiac disease are the leading culprits.) Certain enzymes can also help people with specific digestive problems such as lactose intolerance, bloating, and gas. For the rest of us, however, the supplements appear to be completely unnecessary and have no scientifically verified effect.

What They Are; How They Work

Enzymes are catalysts for virtually every biological and chemical reaction in the body, and digestive enzymes are crucial for the breakdown of food into nutrients the body can absorb. Without sufficient digestive enzymes, the fat, starch, and sugar that we eat can't be fully digested, and this, in turn, can disrupt absorption of minerals and fat-soluble vitamins.

Various digestive enzymes are produced at different points along the digestive tract, from the salivary glands to the small intestine. Other digestive enzymes, including several of the most important, are produced in the pancreas. If the pancreas is chronically infected or damaged by a disease such as cystic fibrosis, the result is severe malabsorption, diarrhea, and malnutrition. In such cases, enzyme supplements can be a lifesaver.

Likewise, if the small intestine fails to produce enough of the digestive enzyme lactase, the milk sugar called lactose will move down the intestinal tract unabsorbed, causing gas, bloating, and diarrhea. A shortage of the enzyme alpha-galactosidase can also have unpleasant consequences, leading to incomplete digestion of certain carbohydrates in foods such as beans and cabbage, and thus causing gas.

Proponents of "enzyme therapy" are not, however, concerned with these specific deficiencies. Instead, they seek to maintain peak digestion by bolstering the body's natural enzymes with ample supplements from other sources. This is thought to reduce the body's workload, allowing the immune system to flourish and ridding the system of toxic, only partially digested nutrients.

How is it that we supposedly lack sufficient enzymes? Many proponents of enzyme therapy blame it on our preference for cooked food. The destruction of enzymes, minerals, and vitamins at the high temperatures used in food preparation is a well-accepted fact. Faced with a shortage of these dietary enzymes, the theory goes, the body's digestive system is forced to compensate by increasing its own enzyme production. Advocates of enzyme therapy hope to ease the extra burden.

Avoid if . . .

According to virtually all medical experts, unless you've been diagnosed with a clear-cut deficiency, enzyme supplements are a waste of money. Clinical research suggests that, for most problems, your odds of success with enzyme therapy are low, while another, more tightly targeted form of treatment might quickly remedy the problem. Be especially wary of experimental cancer treatments with pancreatic enzymes and vitamins A and C. There's no scientific evidence that they do any good.

For people who do suffer an outright deficiency, suppliers warn that pancreatic enzymes cannot be used by those with an allergy to pork protein.

Special Cautions
Digestive Enzyme supplements rarely cause side effects. When problems do occur, they are usually limited to the digestive system. Among the most common are diarrhea, abdominal pain, intestinal obstruction, nausea, vomiting, gas, constipation, and blood in the stool.

Possible Drug Interactions
Pancreatic enzyme supplements available by prescription are not known to interact with other drugs. Enzyme products sold as dietary supplements are said to boost the action of blood-thinning drugs, leading to the need for a dosage adjustment.

Special Information if You Are Pregnant or Breast-feeding
There's no evidence that Digestive Enzyme supplements will cause any harm during pregnancy. Nevertheless, unless you suffer from a serious deficiency, your safest course is to avoid them while pregnant or breast-feeding.

Available Preparations and Dosage
For genuine cases of enzyme deficiency, verified by blood tests and assessment of digestive status, doctors prescribe supplements such as Donnazyme, Cotazyme, Creon, Pancrease, Ultrase, and Zymase. For people with lactose intolerance, there's the over-the-counter remedy Lactaid. And for those troubled by chronic gas, there's a product called Beano.

Enzyme products touted for other disorders are typically sold as dietary supplements. Numerous preparations and combinations are available. Suppliers typically recommend taking from 1 to 4 tablets or capsules before, during, after, or between meals. These products can't legally be sold as a cure for any specific disease. If you're concerned about a particular medical problem, your best bet is to check with your doctor for a more appropriate treatment.

Overdosage
There have been no reports of serious harm.

DMAE (Dimethylaminoethanol)

Why People Take It
DMAE is sold in health food stores as a "brain booster." Its proponents say it enhances memory and learning, increases intelligence, and lifts the mood. Preliminary studies have shown that it lengthens the life span of laboratory animals, although no definitive tests have been conducted on humans.

DMAE's advocates have long claimed that it relieves attention deficit disorder. In addition to improving memory, it is said to decrease aggression in ADD sufferers. From the 1950s until the early 1980s, a prescription drug, Deanol or "deaner," based on DMAE, was prescribed for children suffering from learning disabilities, ADD, and hyperactivity. However, the U.S. Food and Drug Administration forced its withdrawal from the market when a number of studies raised questions about its efficacy.

Promoters claim that DMAE simultaneously aids sleep and improves waking alertness, without the restlessness caused by caffeine. DMAE is also said to decrease anxiety while increasing assertiveness, and it's thought to increase the lucidity of dreams. DMAE also is sold as a hangover remedy, athletic performance booster, and an aid to smoking cessation.

Early studies focused on the possible use of DMAE to relieve trembling caused by long-term use of antipsychotic drugs, but several trials failed to confirm any effectiveness. Attempts to use it as a treatment for Alzheimer's disease also ended in failure. In fact, it was found to actually increase drowsiness and confusion in Alzheimer's patients.

What It Is; How It Works

DMAE is a natural substance found in small amounts in the human brain. It is abundant in fish such as sardines and anchovies—a fact that may have helped to establish the reputation of fish as "brain food."

DMAE's purported memory- and intelligence-enhancing effects are said to stem from its ability to promote the production of acetylcholine, one of the major chemical messengers in the brain. However, not all studies confirm that DMAE is a precursor of acetylcholine, and some medical authorities insist that its mechanism of action is unknown.

Several other actions have been claimed for DMAE. Marketers suggest that it's an efficient antioxidant and free-radical deactivator, and that it strengthens the membranes surrounding the lysosomes. These tiny sacs within the cells collect and digest various toxins and protein-damaging enzymes, and damage to their membranes could result in toxic leakage. DMAE is also said to reverse the formation of lipofuscin, a brown residue of lysosomal digestion that causes so-called aging or liver spots. (This reported effect may account for some of the claims that DMAE fights aging.) DMAE is also said to improve the oxygen capacity of the blood, and to improve the storage life of blood for transfusions.

Proponents of DMAE say that it takes several weeks—or months—for the supplement to make an impact, and that it works better when combined with vitamin B_5 and calcium pantothenate. It is also taken in combination with choline, ginkgo biloba, and other brain stimulants, and is sometimes included in products containing several "brain-boosting" supplements.

Avoid if . . .
People who suffer from a seizure disorder, Alzheimer's disease, or bipolar disorder should not take DMAE.

Special Cautions
DMAE may be overstimulating for some people, and occasionally causes anxiety, nervousness, insomnia, and high blood pressure. A few people may also develop headaches, muscle tension, and leg cramps. Excessive

use increases the likelihood of side effects. Athletes in competition should check the list of banned substances before taking DMAE.

In addition to its use as a dietary supplement, forms of DMAE are marketed as industrial chemicals, used in making dyes, textiles, and emulsifiers in paints and coatings. As an industrial chemical, DMAE is highly corrosive, and appears on government lists of hazardous materials. It may cause adverse effects when inhaled and may be absorbed through the skin. It can irritate the lungs, causing coughing or shortness of breath. Extensive exposure can cause fluid buildup in the lungs, ending in a medical emergency.

Possible Drug Interactions
There are no known drug interactions with DMAE.

Special Information if You Are Pregnant or Breast-feeding
Do not use DMAE while pregnant or breast-feeding.

Available Preparations and Dosage
DMAE is available from a number of suppliers, most commonly in 100-milligram capsules. Manufacturers typically suggest dosages of 1 to 5 capsules per day. Most proponents recommend the lower end of the dosing range, starting with 1 capsule daily. People in their forties and fifties may need 2 capsules a day; older adults may require 3.

Overdosage
Some researchers have used up to 1,600 milligrams of DMAE per day with few reported side effects. However,

the effects of a massive overdose are unknown. If you suspect an overdose, seek medical attention immediately.

DMG (Dimethylglycine)

Why People Take It

This common amino acid derivative has been touted for its immune-boosting and "ergogenic" (energy-enhancing) properties. It has, in fact, been shown to improve the immune response in people exposed to bacterial vaccines. It's also true that it helps promote the use of oxygen in the cells. However, its practical value as an immune-system stimulant and physical energizer has yet to be verified in clinical trials.

Some doctors who specialize in treating children with autism recommend DMG because they have found it to be helpful in some cases. Its effectiveness remains controversial because the only published study in this area suggests that the treatment wasn't effective. However, even the researchers who conducted the trial felt that the dosage and the size of the study were probably too small to be meaningful.

DMG enthusiasts also claim that it can be used to treat epilepsy, headaches, insomnia, memory disorders, heart disease, and the effects of aging. None of these claims has been borne out by any research.

What It Is; How It Works

DMG is a naturally occurring substance found in small amounts in certain foods including brown rice, liver, brewer's yeast, pumpkin seeds, and sesame seeds. It's a derivative of glycine, the most abundant amino acid in the body (see separate entry). It contributes to a number of important biochemical processes in the body, including the respiratory cycle of cells and the regulation of certain hormones.

DMG enhances the immune system by stimulating antibody response and supporting cellular immunity. Promoters of DMG as a food supplement suggest that it may therefore help reverse the gradual decline in immunity brought on by aging, stress, nutritional deficiency, and disease. However, more research is needed to determine exactly how much impact it may have.

Advocates also speculate that, by increasing oxygenation of the tissues, DMG may help boost the body's energy levels. Oxygenation of the muscles, they add, may help to reduce the formation of lactic acid, thus delaying muscle fatigue and improving physical endurance. They also suggest that DMG can supply extra energy during exercise thanks to the role it plays in the production of ATP (adenosine triphosphate), the body's primary cellular fuel. But, like other claims for DMG, all these purported benefits await clinical verification.

Avoid if . . .

As far as researchers know at this point, there are no medical conditions that preclude the use of DMG.

Special Cautions

There has been little research into DMG's safety. Currently, it's thought to be relatively nontoxic and side-effect free.

Possible Drug Interactions

No interactions have been reported. However, DMG is often combined with other ingredients. Read the label to make sure you know what you're taking.

Special Information if You Are Pregnant or Breast-feeding

DMG's safety during this critical period has never been studied. As with any supplement not needed to relieve a serious disorder, your wisest course is to avoid using it during pregnancy and breast-feeding.

Available Preparations and Dosage

There is no official recommended daily intake for DMG. Manufacturers suggest taking 125 to 600 milligrams per day, the larger amount in divided doses.

Overdosage

No reliable information on overdosage is available.

Dolomite

Why People Take It

People take Dolomite for the calcium and magnesium it contains. Along with vitamin D, both these minerals are essential for maintaining strong bones and teeth. Many women now take calcium supplements to stave off the brittle-bone disease osteoporosis.

Although getting extra calcium is an accepted way to lower your risk of osteoporosis, proponents of Dolomite make several other claims that have little scientific support. Dolomite has been promoted as a cleansing agent for teeth, a treatment for inflammation of the bladder, a sleep aid, and a heartbeat regulator. Some researchers have also advanced the theory that the calcium carbonate in Dolomite may discourage the growth of precancerous colon and rectal polyps.

What It Is; How It Works

Dolomite is a natural mineral compound found in especially large deposits in the Dolomite Mountains of northern Italy. It is a calcium magnesium carbonate and, when mined, usually contains at least some traces of other minerals, including potassium and lead. Its lead content has raised serious questions about its safety as a food supplement.

In addition to building bones, the calcium in Dolomite plays a number of other vital roles. It helps muscles to contract, nerves to transmit electrical impulses, and blood to clot. It also strengthens cell membranes and helps regulate the passage of nutrients and other substances in and out of cells. A deficiency leads to muscle cramps, numbness in the arms and legs, weak bones, tooth decay, brittle nails, joint pain, insomnia, and a slow or pounding heartbeat.

The magnesium in Dolomite is equally important for healthy bones: About three-quarters of the body's supply is found in the bones and teeth. It helps the body absorb calcium and other important minerals such as phosphorus, sodium, and potassium. It helps regulate activity of the nerves and muscles, and it activates the enzymes needed for the production of energy. Early warning signs of a deficiency include muscle twitches and tremors, irregular heartbeat, depression, and irritability. Left uncorrected, a deficiency can eventually lead to kidney stones, seizures, and, in extreme cases, diabetic coma.

However, both calcium and magnesium are sufficiently plentiful in most diets to prevent outright deficiencies. And if you do need more, most experts recommend boosting the amount in your diet rather than taking supplements. They say that the body absorbs minerals obtained from food more effectively. Good sources of both minerals include dairy products, the soft bones in canned salmon and sardines, green leafy vegetables, and soy products.

If you do opt for supplementation, Dolomite still may

not be the preferred choice. There are numerous over-the-counter calcium supplements that will meet your calcium needs just as effectively, and some medical experts advise that if magnesium supplements are needed, they should be taken separately from calcium. The close association of the two minerals in the bones may result in one being absorbed at the expense of the other. In addition, extra magnesium is usually needed only under certain special circumstances, such as diabetes, chronic diarrhea, Crohn's disease, and chronic abuse of alcohol.

Avoid if . . .
People with cancer, an overactive parathyroid gland, sarcoidosis, or a tendency to develop kidney stones should check with their doctor before taking any form of supplemental calcium.

Special Cautions
The U.S. Food and Drug Administration and other medical authorities strongly warn against use of Dolomite to meet mineral needs because of its possible lead content. Others note the possibility of lead contamination, but insist that brand-name products are safe.

Possible Drug Interactions
The calcium carbonate in Dolomite may interact with iron preparations such as Feosol and quinolone antibiotics such as Cipro.

Special Information if You Are Pregnant or Breast-feeding
Dolomite could be harmful when taken by women who are pregnant or breast-feeding. An analysis of 70 brands

of calcium supplements found that about a quarter of them exceeded the FDA's total allowable lead intake level for children aged 6 and under. Dolomite was among the highest in lead content.

Available Preparations and Dosage

The recommended dietary intake of calcium ranges from 400 milligrams for infants to 1,500 milligrams for post-menopausal women (who are at greatest risk of osteoporosis). The recommended dietary intake of magnesium is 300 milligrams for adult women and 350 milligrams for adult males.

There is no comparable figure for Dolomite. It is available in tablet form in doses of 250 to 800 milligrams of combined calcium and magnesium. However, because of the FDA warning, few manufacturers still produce or promote it.

Overdosage

The body can generally tolerate up to 2,000 milligrams of calcium daily, although that is more than is needed. Beyond that, calcium can build up in deposits that lead to kidney stones and hardening of the arteries.

A magnesium overdose may result in nausea, vomiting, diarrhea, weakness, low blood pressure, irregular heartbeat, and, in extreme cases, kidney failure.

Fish Oil

Why People Take It

Fish Oil is one of those nutritional megastars that hold promise for a wide variety of chronic conditions. Rich in two omega-3 fatty acids (see separate entry), it may help protect against heart disease, high blood pressure, and some types of cancer. Proponents say the acids could also be useful in the treatment of arthritis, endometriosis, obesity, osteoporosis, and several emotional disorders.

What It Is; How It Works

The two omega-3 fatty acids contained in Fish Oils are eicosapentaenoic acid (EPA) and docosahexaenoic acid (DHA). These acids are especially prevalent in oily cold-water fish such as cod, tuna, mackerel, herring, and salmon. Because the omega-3s come from algae that are then eaten by krill that in turn are eaten by larger fish, farm-raised fish that have been fed grain alone may contain little or none of these beneficial acids.

Omega-3s are thought to protect against heart disease by lowering total cholesterol and triglyceride levels, raising "good" HDL cholesterol, and thinning the blood. They lower the level of fibrinogen, the blood-clotting factor, and keep blood platelets from becoming too sticky, all of which helps to prevent the buildup of artery-clogging plaque. They also tend to dilate the blood vessels, which can help to lower blood pressure in those with hypertension. Recent studies suggest that these beneficial effects of Fish Oil may help reduce the risk of sudden cardiac death, but conclusive proof of this remains lacking.

Some researchers have found that the omega-3s have anti-inflammatory properties that could make them useful in the treatment of arthritis, lupus, and endometriosis. In addition, laboratory experiments suggest that these fatty acids may have an anticancer effect. Other studies indicate that they may help regulate mood in bipolar disorder, depression, schizophrenia, and other psychiatric disorders. And there's even research hinting at a beneficial effect on bone formation, which would make them useful in the treatment and prevention of osteoporosis. They are also being studied for a variety of other disorders, including eczema, psoriasis, and Raynaud's phenomenon.

To obtain the greatest heart benefits from the fatty acids found in fish and fish oils, you need to follow a low-fat diet.

Avoid if . . .
Because of their blood-thinning effects, you should not take Fish Oil supplements if you have a bleeding disorder such as hemophilia or a tendency to hemorrhage.

Special Cautions
Cod liver oil and other fish liver oils are very high in vitamins A and D. Check with your doctor before taking

high doses of these oils, especially if you're taking other vitamin supplements. Dangerously toxic levels could result.

Keep in mind, too, that high doses of these oils sometimes cause an increase in "bad" LDL cholesterol levels. If you have diabetes, you should also be aware that Fish Oil has occasionally been linked to an increase in blood sugar levels.

Potential side effects of Fish Oil capsules include a fishy odor or taste, digestive upset, increased bleeding, and easy bruising. In some people, Fish Oil supplements may negatively affect the immune system.

Possible Drug Interactions
If you are taking a blood-thinning drug such as aspirin or Coumadin, check with your doctor before taking Fish Oil supplements, which could further thin the blood.

Special Information if You Are Pregnant or Breast-feeding
High doses of vitamin A (25,000 IU or more) can cause birth defects, so taking vitamin A–rich cod liver oil during pregnancy is not recommended.

Available Preparations and Dosage
Fish Oil is available in liquid, gel cap, or capsule form. Most Fish Oil supplements range in potency from 200 to 400 milligrams of omega-3 acids. Choose preparations that contain vitamin E to prevent oxidation of the easily damaged oil, and take a little extra vitamin E to prevent oxidation within the body. Supplements that contain 18 percent EPA and 12 percent DHA are generally con-

sidered standard. Pay attention to expiration dates and
refrigerate after opening. Be aware that some preparations may contain pesticides.

There is no recommended dietary allowance (RDA) for
omega-3 fatty acids. Most nutritionists recommend eating
fish 2 or 3 times a week to boost your intake, rather than
taking large amounts of supplements. A 7-ounce serving
of salmon or bluefish provides 2.4 grams of omega-3
acids. The same amount of herring contains 3.2 grams.

Overdosage
High doses taken for a long time can bring on vitamin A
toxicity, with symptoms such as hair loss, headache,
menstrual problems, stiffness, joint pain, weakness, and
dry skin. Vitamin D toxicity, which can lead to irreversible kidney and cardiovascular damage, is also a
danger.

Flaxseed Oil

Why People Take It
Flaxseed Oil has gained attention recently as a potential
alternative to fish oil for prevention of heart disease.
It appears to lower cholesterol, thus discouraging the

buildup of fatty plaque in the arteries. However, unlike fish oil, it does not reduce the high triglyceride levels that may also contribute to heart problems.

Researchers suspect that Flaxseed Oil has anti-inflammatory properties as well, and in at least one clinical study, it has proven to be an effective remedy for symptoms of an enlarged prostate (benign prostatic hyperplasia). Some studies also suggest a beneficial effect on high blood pressure.

What It Is; How It Works

Flaxseed Oil is one of the few vegetable oils that contain alpha linolenic acid. To a limited extent, this compound is converted by the body into EPA (eicosapentaenoic acid), one of the heart-friendly omega-3 oils supplied by fish. EPA, in turn, serves as raw material for a set of chemicals (prostaglandins) that combat inflammation.

Although Flaxseed Oil may keep cholesterol levels in check, it doesn't pack the same punch as fish oil. Some experts suggest that you need to take ten times as much to achieve the same effects. It's also important to avoid confusing the oil with other Flaxseed preparations (cracked, crushed, or milled seeds), which are used to relieve constipation and soothe inflammation of the digestive tract.

Avoid if . . .

There are no medical conditions that preclude the use of Flaxseed Oil.

Special Cautions

Taken in recommended amounts, Flaxseed Oil is unlikely to cause side effects.

Possible Drug Interactions

Flaxseed may delay absorption of drugs taken at the same time.

Special Information if You Are Pregnant or Breast-feeding

At normal dosage levels, no harmful effects are known. Nevertheless, it's best to check with your doctor before taking this or any other supplement during this critical period.

Available Preparations and Dosage

Flaxseed Oil is available in liquid and capsule form. Daily doses of 1 tablespoonful or 5 capsules are typical. Because the size of the capsules varies, follow the manufacturer's instructions unless otherwise advised by your doctor.

Overdosage

No information is available.

Fructo-Oligosaccharides (FOS)

Why People Take Them

Though your taste buds recognize them as sugar, Fructo-Oligosaccharides (FOS) have one extra molecule that makes them too large for humans to digest. Instead, they fuel the growth of the beneficial bacteria that reside in everyone's intestines. These microorganisms protect against infections and—perhaps—reduce the risk of gastrointestinal cancers. Proponents also credit FOS with increasing the absorption of calcium, lowering blood sugar and cholesterol levels, and relieving constipation, diarrhea, vaginitis, mouth ulcers (canker sores), indigestion, and heartburn.

What They Are; How They Work

Fructo-Oligosaccharides are sometimes referred to as prebiotics, since they promote the growth of probiotics—the good bacteria like *L. acidophilus* and *B. bifidum* that maintain intestinal health. (Interestingly, bad bacteria, such as *E. coli*, are unable to make use of FOS.)

Also known as inulin or neosugar, Fructo-Oligosaccharides are naturally occurring sugars found in many foods, including bananas, barley, garlic, honey, onions, wheat, and tomatoes. Fresh Jerusalem artichokes are a particularly good source of FOS, but nutritional supplements provide them in an even more concentrated form. Because they are not digested, when you consume FOS your blood sugar levels remain stable.

For optimal health, the body must maintain the right balance between good and bad bacteria. As we age, the number of good bacteria declines. FOS supplements reverse this trend. Studies have shown that when they're taken by older people, their *Bifidobacterium* count rises. There's also a decrease in the pH (which translates to an increase in the acidity) of the lower intestine, making it inhospitable to bad bacteria. And Japanese studies have shown that adding 3 to 6 grams of FOS to the daily diet can reduce the level of toxic cancer-causing compounds in human waste by over 40 percent within three weeks

Avoid if . . .
FOS appears to be safe for everyone.

Special Cautions
Fructo-Oligosaccharides are not toxic and are free of side effects.

Possible Drug Interactions
No interactions have been reported.

Special Information if You Are Pregnant or Breast-feeding
There's no reason to believe that FOS would cause any harm. As with any supplement, however, it's best to check with your doctor before taking them.

Available Preparations and Dosage

Some companies sell FOS as a nutritional supplement, while others add it to their probiotics. It's available in capsules and powder which can be mixed into liquids. Probiotic enthusiasts generally recommend 4 to 8 grams per day. Start with 1 gram daily. If you have a chronic yeast infection, gas, bloating, or other digestive problems, you may want to increase your dose to 4 grams daily.

Overdosage

While the maximum recommended daily dosage of FOS is 18 grams, no amount appears to cause toxicity.

GABA (Gamma-Aminobutyric Acid)

Why People Take It

Nerve cells pass along messages by firing brief bursts of chemicals (neurotransmitters) into receptor sites on adjacent cells. GABA is one of these neurotransmitters. But unlike some of the other chemical messengers in the brain, this one tends to *inhibit* further transmissions instead of triggering them. It has a stabilizing effect on brain cells, preventing them from firing too fast or too frequently. Studies show that an inadequate or disrupted GABA supply is associated with disorders such as anxiety, insomnia, epilepsy, premenstrual syndrome (PMS), pain, and possibly depression.

Ever since GABA's role in maintaining a healthy biochemical balance in the brain was established, pharmaceutical manufacturers have sought to develop drugs that mimic its action. Several prescription medications that seem to affect GABA activity or GABA receptor sites in the brain are now on the market and are used to reduce anxiety, relieve pain, induce sleep, or control seizures. New GABA-related compounds are being studied and new uses are being found for them all the time. Recent studies show that these agents may also be useful in treating PMS and gastroesophageal reflux disease (GERD).

The synthetic GABA supplements found in health food stores are, however, a different matter. Their manufacturers claim that these products augment the brain's natural GABA supply and stabilize its effects. But the consequences of taking GABA supplements, if any, are still unknown. And some experts have even questioned the body's ability to absorb and make use of GABA in the form found in such supplements.

Still, GABA's promoters continue to tout it as the "Valium" of nutritional supplements. In addition to claiming a relaxant effect, some manufacturers promote GABA to increase sex drive, treat enlarged prostate, and relieve attention deficit disorder. Marketers of bodybuilding supplements claim that GABA can also be used to decrease body fat and enhance athletic performance by stimulating growth hormone production. Though these claims are enticing, none has been scientifically verified.

What It Is; How It Works

GABA is an amino acid compound produced in the body from glutamic acid. It is one of the most abundant neurotransmitters in the brain. Although GABA activity is affected by other substances in the brain such as enzymes and hormones, scientists don't fully understand how GABA levels get out of balance. They do know, however, that sufficient levels of GABA must be maintained to ensure equilibrium in the system—and that there is a delicate balance between too much stimulation and too little.

Producers of manufactured GABA, on the other hand, seem to operate on the assumption that if a little is good, more will be better. They argue that taking a supplement when natural supplies are low is bound to produce beneficial effects. At this point, however, this theory hasn't been tested and we don't know if it's true.

Avoid if . . .

There are no known conditions precluding the use of GABA supplements.

Special Cautions

If you are taking a prescription medication for epilepsy, anxiety, or insomnia, don't abruptly discontinue it when you start taking GABA; serious problems could develop. For safety's sake, check with your doctor before using GABA for these and other medical conditions.

Possible Drug Interactions

There are no reported drug interactions with GABA, but some researchers suspect combining GABA supplements with tranquilizers such as Valium or Xanax could lead to heightened effects. Taking GABA with alcohol is also not recommended.

Special Information if You Are Pregnant or Breast-feeding
The safety of GABA supplementation during pregnancy has not been verified. Your safest course is to avoid it while pregnant or breast-feeding.

Available Preparations and Dosage
GABA is available in capsule form in strengths varying from 100 to 750 milligrams. Some manufacturers suggest taking 500 to 1000 milligrams a day, the higher amount divided into smaller doses. (Beware, however: One source advises against taking more than 500 milligrams a day.) When using GABA for insomnia, take it at bedtime.

Overdosage
While no information on overdose is available, high doses of GABA are reported to cause agitation and *increase* anxiety, as well as cause numbness around the mouth and tingling in the arms and legs.

Gelatin

Why People Take It

As any reader of health and beauty magazines knows, gelatin is a popular remedy for poor hair and nails. Whatever its actual benefits, it has enjoyed this reputation for generations. Lately, however, Gelatin has sparked interest for an entirely different reason. Among arthritis sufferers it is now discussed along with chondroitin and glucosamine as a "natural" approach to treating joint pain and joint disease.

What It Is; How It Works

Gelatin, while often called a natural product, cannot be found in nature. It is manufactured by boiling skin, tendons, ligaments, and bones taken from cows and pigs. The end product is a mixture of animal proteins, including several amino acids (glycine, proline, and hydroxyproline). When dry, Gelatin is a tasteless powder. When mixed with liquid, it forms a gel used throughout the food and pharmaceutical industries. It serves as a stabilizer and thickener in confectionery and ice cream, and provides the raw material for the capsules used for many medicines. It is classified by the U.S. Food and Drug Administration as a "generally recognized as safe" food additive.

Gelatin is an inexpensive source of animal protein. But that protein is incomplete, lacking the essential amino acid tryptophan and offering only small amounts of some others. Its value in maintaining joint health is subject to debate. Proponents say it provides large amounts of two amino acids (proline and glycine) that the body uses to make collagen, an important part of joint cartilage. But since these two amino acids are manufactured by the body as needed, and no shortage has been documented in cases of joint disease, the basis for any benefits from supplementation remains unclear.

Proponents of Gelatin cite a handful of studies as evidence of its effectiveness. One trial, funded by a manufacturer, found that gelatin reduced joint pain and improved flexibility among the twenty athletes in the eight-week study. The researchers argued that the amino acids in Gelatin promote cartilage development, and that increased consumption gives the joints more raw materials to use for repair. A more demanding trial was conducted in 1985 on 51 people with arthritis in their hips and knees. The half of the group using Gelatin therapeutically for two months experienced less pain but were no more mobile than the half using a placebo (dummy treatment).

Most experts consider these and other studies too small and too limited to provide any conclusive answers about Gelatin's benefits. Gelatin seems to do no harm and may be helpful to some people, but there's no evidence that it can cure arthritis by itself. Even if you take it, you should consult your doctor for other—possibly more effective—treatments.

Avoid if . . .
Side effects are rare, but allergic reactions to Gelatin have
been reported. If you suffer from food allergies, proceed
with caution. Since Gelatin is an animal product, vegetarians will want to avoid it.

Special Cautions
Because Gelatin is produced from cattle, there is a danger
that it could carry bovine spongiform encephalopathy
(BSE), also known as mad cow disease. The FDA has
banned the import for food and pharmaceutical use of
any Gelatin from countries where BSE is present in the
cattle population. However, the FDA does not regulate
dietary supplements, so Gelatin sold as a supplement is
not subject to the ban. If you are concerned about possible transmission of BSE, you should check with the
supplement's manufacturer to determine the source of the
Gelatin, or forgo taking it.

Possible Drug Interactions
No drug interactions are known.

Special Information if You Are Pregnant or Breast-feeding
No problems during pregnancy have been reported.
Nevertheless, it's wise to double check with your doctor
before taking any supplement.

Available Preparations and Dosage
Plain Gelatin is readily available in grocery stores, health
food stores, and pharmacies in capsule, tablet, and powdered form. The pills typically contain 650 milligrams of
Gelatin. Recommended dosages have not been estab-

lished. Follow the manufacturer's instructions or check
with your doctor.

Overdosage
No information on overdosage is available.

Germanium

Why People Take It
Germanium first entered the health-and-fitness spotlight
in the 1970s, after a Japanese scientist announced that it
could relieve rheumatoid arthritis, cure certain forms
of cancer, and protect against a host of degenerative disorders. It is still promoted for these problems today, and
is now sold as a treatment for high blood pressure and
high cholesterol as well. It is said to have both antioxidant properties and an antiviral effect. Lately it has
received attention as a potential remedy for osteoporosis
and Alzheimer's disease.

There's good reason to think twice, however, before
experimenting with this substance. Although it is available over the counter and can be found in a number of
foods and herbs, it's the subject of a U.S. Food and Drug
Administration (FDA) hazard assessment declaring that
"Germanium products present a potential human health

hazard." When cases of kidney failure, and even death, occurred following its use, the FDA imposed a ban on imports and forced certain Germanium products off the market.

Manufacturers insist that some forms of *organic* Germanium (Ge-132, germanium-lactate-citrate, and others) are safe even at high dosages. Promoters of organic Germanium as a supplement argue that it has been extensively studied and found to be "virtually nontoxic," and they object to being associated with the hazardous form, *inorganic* Germanium (germanium dioxide). However, there is at least one reported incident of irreversible kidney damage after use of one of the so-called safe substances; and the FDA hazard warning on Germanium applies to both the inorganic *and* organic forms, especially when used for prolonged periods of time.

What It Is; How It Works

Germanium is a trace element found in both plants and animals. Some medical authorities argue that it's an essential part of the diet, while others disagree. A normal diet supplies an estimated daily intake of between 0.5 and 3.5 milligrams. No one has ever shown evidence of a deficiency. Foods rich in Germanium include garlic, onions, shiitake mushrooms, ginseng, and comfrey.

Germanium owes its popularity to the Japanese scientist Kazuhiko Asai. Dr. Asai noticed that many Asian herbal remedies contained higher-than-usual amounts of Germanium, as did the healing waters at Lourdes. He theorized that most disease processes originate from an acid excess caused by oxygen deprivation in the blood. He believed that Germanium could help correct this imbalance by removing excess hydrogen and improving oxygen delivery. After years of experimentation with various forms, he developed the organic Germanium formula known as Ge-132 and pronounced it a miracle cure and preventive for illness.

There is no shortage of research on the organic forms of Germanium, though very little work has been done in humans. In tests on laboratory animals, organic Germanium has been found to stimulate an immune response by inducing interferon production and activating natural killer cells. These agents of the immune system are part of the body's line of defense against diseases such as cancer, as indicated by another study in which a Germanium compound blocked the progression of lung cancer in mice. In yet another animal study, researchers showed that treating mice with organic Germanium appeared to prevent the accumulation of the cellular debris that is associated with Alzheimer's disease. And scientists examining the effects of organic Germanium on mice with induced osteoporosis have found that Ge-132 prevents the decrease in bone density and bone strength caused by osteoporosis.

While Germanium's exact mechanism of action is still unknown, supporters speculate that many of the research results obtained with lab animals stem from the compound's ability to improve oxygenation of the tissues. (Some promoters package Germanium as "vitamin O," for oxygen.) Germanium is also said to have a significant impact on the immune system, boosting synthesis of the antiviral substance interferon, activating the large killer cells called macrophages, and stimulating production of T-suppressor cells.

Avoid if . . .
Do not take Germanium if you have any kind of kidney or liver disorder.

Special Cautions
Since there is very little regulation of dietary supplements, you can't be certain about the quality and purity of over-the-counter Germanium. Buy only from a source you trust, and see your doctor regularly to be monitored for toxic effects. (Industrial-grade germanium used as an electrical semiconductor is considered toxic and should never be ingested.)

Prolonged use of Germanium products can lead to kidney failure and even death. Signs of Germanium toxicity include yellow skin and eyes, digestive upsets, fatigue, gastrointestinal bleeding, anemia, muscle weakness, and nerve pain.

Possible Drug Interactions
There are no known drug interactions associated with Germanium.

Special Information if You Are Pregnant or Breast-feeding
Given its possible toxicity, Germanium should be strictly avoided during pregnancy and breast-feeding.

Available Preparations and Dosage
Organic Germanium is available in powder and capsule form. Strengths range from 25 to 150 milligrams. There is no recommended dietary intake for Germanium. Because of the serious health risks associated with its use, check with your doctor before taking it.

Overdosage

While there are no reports of acute toxicity from a single massive overdose of Germanium, remember that long-term use of Germanium supplements may lead to kidney and liver damage.

GLA (Gamma-Linolenic Acid)

Why People Take It

Gamma-Linolenic Acid (GLA) is a fatty acid that the body uses to produce hormonelike substances called prostaglandins—particularly "prostaglandin E1." This type of prostaglandin fights inflammation, and GLA is often used to treat the inflammation and pain of arthritis. Some studies have found that it provides relief, particularly for rheumatoid arthritis, but not all test results have been positive. Preparations containing GLA are also used to treat a variety of symptoms associated with premenstrual syndrome (PMS) and may be helpful for some people with eczema.

GLA is one of the more thoroughly studied natural substances. It is generally regarded as essential to healthy skin, hair, and nails. It has been shown to enhance the immune system in older adults. It also increases "good" prostaglandins and decreases the "bad" ones that can lead to hardening of the arteries, prompting some researchers to speculate that it could be helpful in preventing or treating heart disease. There is also some evidence that GLA can lower total cholesterol and improve "good" cholesterol levels.

In addition to rheumatoid arthritis, GLA may relieve other inflammatory autoimmune conditions such as Sjögren's syndrome (chronically dry eyes and mouth). Studies on a painful degenerative nerve condition suffered by diabetics, who can't process GLA properly, found that supplements provided relief. Oils containing GLA have proven helpful for people hospitalized with acute respiratory distress syndrome.

GLA's promoters have also claimed it can be used to treat cancer, schizophrenia, childhood hyperactivity, irritable bowel syndrome, endometriosis, multiple sclerosis, lupus, Raynaud's disease, and the repetitive involuntary movements dubbed tardive dyskinesia. There is little scientific evidence to support these claims and, for some conditions, such as tardive dyskinesia, research has found that GLA seems to have no effect.

What It Is; How It Works
The body manufactures its own supply of Gamma-Linolenic Acid from linolenic acid, one of the essential fatty acids we obtain from our diets. However, due to disease, dietary imbalance, or the effects of aging, some people either cannot manufacture GLA from linolenic acid or can't convert GLA into prostaglandins. Such people are candidates for GLA supplementation. Rich sources are oils from evening primrose, borage, and black currant seeds.

Some nutritional experts have recently suggested that Americans may be suffering from a widespread deficiency of essential fatty acids such as linolenic acid. At one time in our history, daily intake of potentially harmful saturated fats was about equal to that of the beneficial polyunsaturated fats. Under those conditions, enough of the raw material to manufacture GLA, and thus prostaglandins, was taken in through a normal diet.

However, during the last century daily fat intake has not only increased sharply, but has also included a growing amount of unhealthy hydrogenated oils and trans fatty acids. Today, the ratio of saturated to polyunsaturated dietary fats stands at about six to one, and many experts believe that the relative lack of essential fatty acids has combined with the hyperabundance of saturated fats and hydrogenated oils to promote clogged arteries and heart disease while reducing production of potentially protective GLA.

Avoid if . . .
There is no known reason to avoid GLA supplements.

Special Cautions
Be sure to get adequate amounts of magnesium, zinc, vitamin C, and the B vitamins when taking GLA. Some nutritional experts believe these nutrients are needed to support conversion of GLA to prostaglandin E1.

Possible Drug Interactions
No interactions are known.

Special Information if You Are Pregnant or Breast-feeding
GLA is not known to be harmful. However, as with any supplement, it's wise to check with your doctor before taking it during this critical period.

Available Preparations and Dosage
Researchers studying GLA have typically used daily doses of 150 to 300 milligrams, although some studies have been done with 250 to 500 milligrams. The total daily intake is divided into smaller doses. It may take 6 to 8 weeks for results to appear.

The three major sources of GLA—evening primrose, borage, and black currant seed oil—are available in capsules or softgels (gel caps), which vary in the amount they supply. A 500-milligram capsule of evening primrose oil contains between 35 and 45 milligrams of GLA. The same-sized capsule of borage oil contains about 120 milligrams of GLA. Black currant seed oil has about 80 milligrams of GLA per 500-milligram capsule.

Overdosage
No information on overdosage is available.

Glandular Extracts

Why People Take Them

Taking a cue from homeopathic medicine—which rests on the Greek adage of "Like cures like"—advocates of these supplements believe that preparations made from animal glands can be used to jump-start poorly functioning human glands. Bodybuilders and athletes in particular think they can gain an edge by taking glandular extracts. Likewise, some people use them in an attempt to strengthen their immune system. For example, those with AIDS and those with rheumatoid arthritis use glandular extracts in the hopes of curing their disease, while others use them to battle chronic infections like hepatitis. But despite minor changes observed in some lab results, the majority of evidence provides little reason to expect any therapeutic benefit from these products.

Glandular extracts have also been promoted as a weapon against aging. Some proponents say that because our bodies produce fewer hormones as we age, animal-based glandular products can help slow down, and maybe even reverse, the aging process. However, though the theory is alluring, there's no real-world evidence to support it.

139

It's important to distinguish over-the-counter glandular extracts from the hormonal medications that play such a vital role in modern medicine. The insulin used for diabetes, the thyroid hormone prescribed for a sluggish metabolism, and the steroids used to reduce pain and inflammation are all products of various glands. But unlike store-bought glandular extracts, these medications, in the right doses, have a well-established track record for unquestionable efficacy.

What It Is; How It Works

Extracts can be found for just about any gland, including the thyroid, liver, thymus, pancreas, and adrenals. These preparations are made from the glands of animals, usually pigs or cows, and supposedly stimulate activity in similar tissues. For example, thymus extract is intended to prompt the thymus gland into producing more antibodies, thereby strengthening the immune system. (Results of experiments with thymus extract have been mixed, with some studies showing moderate improvement in some patients, and other studies finding nothing.)

Proponents also speculate that glandular supplements promote "conservation"—that is, taking a particular extract will spare the corresponding gland from extra work. However, the mechanism that allows this to happen has never been established. (If it did happen, stopping a supplement could prove dangerous, since glandular activity might be slow to return to normal.)

Some scientists question whether the body can actually absorb oral supplements made from animal glands, although recent studies conclude that, in theory at least, a small amount could reach the bloodstream. On the other hand, the efficacy of certain glandular supplements in the digestive tract is undisputed. Enzymes taken to supplement the output of an underperforming pancreas act within the intestines, and yield an immediate improvement in digestion. Speculation that these enzymes can also relieve immune disorders remains to be verified, however; and there's no proof that they have any value in cancer therapy.

Avoid if . . .

A variety of medical problems can be corrected with authentic hormone therapy, but establishing the correct dosage is a complex matter that requires appropriate medical tests and supervision by your doctor. Truly effective products are generally available only by prescription. Self-medicating with over-the-counter extracts—if it has any effect at all—could throw your delicately balanced hormone system out of kilter. If you suspect any sort of glandular problem, don't waste valuable time experimenting with these products. Instead, make an appointment with your doctor.

Special Cautions

Short-term side effects from taking one of these extracts can range from stomach upset to loss of feeling and tingling in the limbs. Long-term side effects are unknown.

Before taking any glandular product, it's wise to check the source. The U.S. Food and Drug Administration has concerns that imported extracts could be contaminated with the same proteins that cause the rare form of brain degeneration known as "mad cow disease."

Possible Drug Interactions

It is not known whether glandular extracts interact with medications. If you've been prescribed any medication on a regular basis, check with your doctor before taking an extract.

Special Information if You Are Pregnant or Breast-feeding

Glandular extracts should *never* be taken during pregnancy or while breast-feeding.

Available Preparations and Dosage

Some proponents of glandular extracts believe that predigested, water-soluble forms are the most effective. Practitioners of naturopathic medicine caution that such extracts should be used only for a short time, since the gland should continue to function on its own after receiving this jump start.

Dosage varies according to both the type of extract and its form of preparation. Follow the manufacturer's directions and check with a doctor if you have any doubts. The supplements should be stored in a cool, dry place, but should not be frozen. Store them safely away from children.

Overdosage

No information on overdosage is available.

Glucosamine

Why People Take It

Although this natural remedy still inspires controversy, it has gained increasing acceptance as a treatment for the joint pain and inflammation of osteoarthritis. Many advocates say that it may also slow progression of the disease.

Because of its ability to reduce and—in some cases—completely eliminate the pain of osteoarthritis, some physicians and researchers feel Glucosamine might offer similar benefits for people suffering from rheumatoid arthritis, ankylosing spondylitis, spinal disc degeneration, tendinitis, bursitis, and physical injuries to the joints. There is even speculation that it could play a preemptive role, eliminating the development of osteoarthritis in people over 40.

What It Is; How It Works

Glucosamine is a natural sugar produced by the body and found in certain foods. It plays an important role in the production, maintenance, and repair of cartilage, the white, smooth, rubberlike padding that covers the ends of bones and prevents them from rubbing against each other painfully as we move. It also helps form ligaments, tendons, and nails.

Glucosamine stimulates the production of glycosaminoglycans and proteoglycans, two essential building blocks of cartilage. In most cases, the joints produce sufficient Glucosamine to keep the cartilage in good repair, but if they fail to do so, it dries out, degenerates, cracks, and may even completely wear away. Left unprotected, the joints then become swollen, stiff, inflamed, tender, and painful—the condition known as osteoarthritis.

While Glucosamine has been used to treat osteoarthritis in Europe since the 1980s, its use in the United States has been confined mainly to arthritic animals. However, several scientific studies have recently supported its effectiveness, and its popularity in this country is spreading quickly. There's also a widely held—but unproven—theory that combining Glucosamine with chondroitin sulfate increases its effectiveness.

Avoid if . . .
No known medical conditions preclude the use of Glucosamine.

Special Cautions
Although Glucosamine may relieve your osteoarthritis, other treatments, such as a regular exercise program, remain just as important. If you have this condition, it's wise to keep in touch with your doctor for regular checkups.

Unlike the potent nonsteroidal anti-inflammatory drugs (NSAIDs) usually prescribed for arthritis, Glucosamine does not produce serious side effects. You might, however, experience mild symptoms such as diarrhea, heartburn, indigestion, and nausea. Try taking the medication with food if it upsets your stomach (or if you have an ulcer). If this fails to eliminate the symptoms, check with your doctor.

Possible Drug Interactions
Glucosamine sulfate taken alone or in combination with chondroitin does not interfere with NSAIDs, aspirin, or any other anti-inflammatory or analgesic medication. Indeed, there is some evidence that taking this supplement may help people reduce their use of these strong drugs.

Special Information if You Are Pregnant or Breast-feeding
Check with your doctor before taking Glucosamine while pregnant or breast-feeding.

Available Preparations and Dosage
Glucosamine is available in three forms:

Glucosamine sulfate. This is considered the preparation of choice for osteoarthritis.
Glucosamine hydrochloride. This is the least expensive variety. It is used primarily for arthritic animals.
N-acetyl glucosamine. This form delivers less of the active ingredient to the joints.

Glucosamine sulfate capsules and Glucosamine sulfate–chondroitin combination capsules and tablets can be found in many health food stores and may also be ordered by mail.

There is no consensus on the ideal dosage of

Glucosamine sulfate. Some doctors recommend 1,000 to 2,000 milligrams per day. Others suggest up to 3,000 milligrams per day, since they insist it is safe and produces no serious side effects. Dosage can be adjusted according to your response. If you are overweight or are taking a water pill (diuretic), you may need a higher dosage.

Some people experience pain relief immediately. Nevertheless, it may take anywhere from 8 weeks to 6 months to repair damaged cartilage.

Overdosage
No information on overdosage is available.

Glutamine

Why People Take It
This common amino acid serves as an energy storehouse. It also supports healthy muscle tissue and provides the intestinal lining with needed fuel. In addition, it's used by the white blood cells that protect the body from infection.

Glutamine supplements are used primarily by four groups:

1. Dedicated athletes, to improve performance and prevent the breakdown of muscle tissue

2. People with weakened immunity, such as AIDS patients, to help prevent wasting and muscle atrophy
3. Those with intestinal conditions such as gastritis, ulcers, and colitis, to help protect the intestinal lining
4. Individuals withdrawing from alcohol

What It Is; How It Works

As the building blocks of human protein, amino acids are a vital part of everyone's diet. Glutamine is the most abundant amino acid in the body, and, as such, is involved in more metabolic processes than any other. It is stored primarily in muscle tissue, then converted to glucose and transported to whatever part of the body requires energy. It is particularly important as a source of fuel for cells lining the intestines. Without it, these cells waste away.

Converted to the related compound glutamate and combined with N-acetylcysteine (see entry on cysteine), it promotes the synthesis of glutathione (see separate entry). The body's major antioxidant, glutathione plays an important role in neutralizing harmful waste products and toxins. Glutathione levels often drop significantly in people with HIV infection, leading to a dangerous condition called HIV wasting syndrome, in which, for some unknown reason, people lose weight and muscle tone. Glutamine or L-glutamine is commonly given to counteract the wasting, and to strengthen immunity in hospital patients who have been weakened by infection or other immune-stressing illnesses.

While the body is capable of manufacturing its own supply of Glutamine, deficiencies can develop during extended fasting, cirrhosis, and weight loss due to AIDS or cancer. High-protein foods, such as most meat and dairy products, provide generous amounts of Glutamine. A variety of Glutamine supplements are also available.

Avoid if . . .
Because excess amino acids can put a strain on the liver and kidneys, it's best to avoid Glutamine if you have kidney or liver problems or are undergoing chemotherapy.

Special Cautions
The most common side effect of Glutamine supplementation is occasional constipation. To prevent it, drink at least 10 glasses of water per day. If you suffer from chronic constipation, you should also supplement your diet with some type of soluble fiber while taking Glutamine.

Possible Drug Interactions
If you are taking antibiotics to cure stomach ulcers, check with your doctor before taking Glutamine. It can interfere with some of these drugs.

Special Information if You Are Pregnant or Breast-feeding
No specific information is available. However, it's wise to check with your doctor before taking any supplement while pregnant or breast-feeding.

Available Preparations and Dosage
Glutamine is available in capsules and as a powder. Doses of up to 20 to 25 grams daily are said to be safe, but experts recommend that you take no more than 1.5 grams daily unless your doctor orders a higher dose.

Since Glutamine is tasteless, it can be mixed with

water in its powder form, but do not add it to hot foods or acidic ones, such as orange juice, since they can change the chemical composition of the supplement.

Overdosage
No information on overdosage is available.

Glutathione

Why People Take It
Glutathione is the body's key line of defense against the harmful oxygen by-products called free radicals. It's also a key player in many of the reactions that neutralize foreign toxins within the body. Proponents claim that Glutathione supplements can help treat lead poisoning and damage from other heavy metals, lower the toxicity of chemotherapy and radiation in cancer patients, reverse cataracts, and prevent oxygen toxicity during hyperbaric oxygen therapy. Others believe that the nutrient may help protect the liver from alcohol-induced damage. Unfortunately, the jury is still out on most of these claims.

There is, however, some scientific evidence to suggest that Glutathione may help people with HIV infection, the cause of AIDS. Clinical trials have shown that Glutathione levels in the body drop during HIV infection, and low levels of Glutathione seem to be linked to poor survival among patients.

Similarly, test-tube experiments have shown that a shortage of Glutathione depresses the function of T lymphocytes, a key group in the immune system's arsenal of infection-fighting agents. That could be important to HIV-positive patients because it is these white blood cells that come under attack in AIDS.

Human studies also hint at the possibility that giving HIV-positive patients a drug like N-acetylcysteine— which the body converts into Glutathione—may help fight the disease. Unfortunately no large-scale scientific studies have yet been done to confirm these preliminary results.

Some researchers also believe that persons who are on kidney dialysis may benefit from Glutathione. In one experiment, 1,200 milligrams of intravenous Glutathione helped control the damage to red blood cells that often accompanies dialysis. The patients' hemoglobin levels improved and their red blood cells became healthier.

What It Is; How It Works

Glutathione is made up of three amino acids: cysteine, glutamic acid, and glycine. (See separate entries.) It's produced naturally by the body and plays an important role in maintaining the health of virtually every cell.

Glutathione's protective role depends partially on its ability to act as an antioxidant. Like vitamins C and E, Glutathione protects cell membranes from the damaging effects of free radicals. Acting as a natural antitoxin, it also helps rid the body of poisonous chemicals. But most of the research that suggests Glutathione supplements can protect us from toxic substances like pesticides or heavy metals was done in animals. And since animal and human physiology are often quite different, there's no way to be sure at this point whether the supplements have the same beneficial effects in humans.

Avoid if . . .
There's no known reason to avoid this nutrient.

Special Cautions
No toxic side effects have been reported.

Possible Drug Interactions
Some doctors have suggested that supplements containing Glutathione should be avoided by cancer patients on radiation or chemotherapy. Some of these treatments partially depend on damaging free radicals to kill cancerous cells, and antioxidants such as Glutathione inhibit the formation of free radicals. Such concerns, however, have been proven unwarranted by further research. In fact, during a British study of 150 women with ovarian cancer who were receiving the anticancer drug cisplatin, those who were also given a fifteen-minute IV infusion of Glutathione not only remained responsive to the cisplatin, but also developed fewer complications from the anticancer drug than did patients given a dummy infusion.

Special Information if You Are Pregnant or Breast-feeding
To date, there are no reports indicating that Glutathione is harmful during pregnancy or breast-feeding. But because the supplement has never been tested for safety during these periods, your safest course is to avoid its use.

Available Preparations and Dosages

There is no recommended dietary allowance for Glutathione, and under normal conditions the body is able to manufacture all it needs from amino acids in the diet. Supplements, however, can be purchased in tablet, capsule, and powder form. Because formulations vary, always follow the manufacturer's dosage instructions.

Overdosage

Glutathione is not known to be toxic at any dosage level, although few tests have been done.

Glycine

Why People Take It

Glycine is one of the many nutritional supplements adopted by bodybuilders to boost physical performance. Its popularity stems from its role in the formation of creatine, a key ingredient in the chemical reaction that powers the muscles. (See separate entry.) Unfortunately, while creatine may indeed enhance performance, Glycine alone does not seem to have the same effect. In fact, the American Dietetic Association notes that Glycine and other supposedly ergogenic (energy-producing) substances may owe their standing more to psychological than to any physical effects.

Over-the-counter Glycine supplements have been touted for a variety of purposes. The substance promotes elimination of the uric acid responsible for gout, and is used as a remedy. It's also said to have a calming effect and, when paired with glutamine, is believed to stave off cravings for alcohol. It's thought to be helpful in decreasing spastic conditions such as epilepsy and multiple sclerosis, and has been used to treat hypoglycemia. Its advocates also say that in high doses (4 to 8 grams), it stimulates the release of growth hormone.

Glycine's proponents assert that it stimulates N-methyl-D-aspartic acid (NMDA) receptors in the brain, thereby enhancing mental function. Based on this assumption, Glycine has been proposed as a treatment for mental disorders such as bipolar disorder and schizophrenia. However, in small clinical trials among people with schizophrenia, it has produced only mixed results.

At least one review of the scientific literature has uncovered substantial experimental evidence that Glycine may have a role in protecting tissues against damaging disruptions of the blood and oxygen supplies. But animal studies have not produced consistent results, and clinical trials have yet to confirm a protective effect.

Glycine appears naturally in prostate fluid, and is used as a bladder irrigation solution during transurethral resection of the prostate (TURP) and other surgeries involving the urinary canal.

What It Is; How It Works

Glycine is one of the "nonessential" amino acids that the body can produce for itself whenever they fall short in the diet. It's also available from high-protein foods such as meat, fish, beans, and dairy products.

Glycine combines with two other amino acids—arginine and methionine—to build energy-producing creatine. It also promotes the storage of blood sugar (glucose) in the form of glycogen. Together with the amino acids cysteine and glutamic acid, it produces the protective antioxidant glutathione (see separate entry). It plays an important role in the production of oxygen-carrying hemoglobin, and in the synthesis of nucleic acid. On top of all these duties, it also serves as one of the nervous system's chemical messengers, inhibiting neuro-logical responses in the spinal cord.

Avoid if . . .

High doses of Glycine and other amino acids lay an extra burden on the liver and kidneys. If you have a problem in either area, don't take Glycine without your doctor's approval.

Special Cautions

When used as an irrigation solution in transurethral sur-geries, Glycine has caused side effects such as excessive urination, urinary retention, high or low blood pressure, backache, nausea, vomiting, swelling, thirst, and dehy-dration. However, studies conducted with oral Glycine supplements have encountered no such problems.

Possible Drug Interactions
There are no reported interactions.

Special Information if You Are Pregnant or Breast-feeding
It's not known whether high levels of Glycine are safe during pregnancy. As with any supplement not absolutely necessary for your health, it's best to avoid Glycine while pregnant or breast-feeding.

Available Preparations and Dosage
Glycine is available in tablet, capsule, and powder form in doses ranging from 100 to 600 milligrams. There is no recommended dietary allowance for glycine. Follow the manufacturer's directions closely.

Overdosage
Reportedly, high doses can cause fatigue. If you suspect an overdose, check with your doctor.

Glycosaminoglycans (GAGs)

Why People Take Them
Hardening and clogging of the arteries (atherosclerosis) is widely known as a major cause of heart disease and stroke. It takes hold when high blood pressure, cigarette

smoking, or other factors damage the inner lining of blood vessels, creating rough patches that snag cholesterol and debris.

Glycosaminoglycans (GAGs) form part of the structure the body uses to reinforce blood-vessel walls, and preliminary evidence suggests that they may be helpful in slowing the progress of a variety of vascular disorders, including atherosclerosis, varicose veins, phlebitis, and hemorrhoids. And when blood pressure is under control, GAGs may also prevent kidney problems in people with type 2 diabetes (the kind that usually doesn't require insulin shots).

What They Are; How They Work

GAGs, which are needed to make cartilage and build strong connective tissue, are found throughout the body, including the joints and the lining of blood vessels. While they are very important, GAGs are not considered "essential" nutrients because the body usually manufactures them from scratch. Chondroitin (see separate entry), a major component of cartilage and a popular arthritis remedy, is a type of GAG. Unlike chondroitin, however, GAG supplements are used primarily to treat diseases of blood vessels.

GAGs are long chains of sugars—including glucosamine, chondroitin, and heparin—attached to a core protein. The whole entity, which is shaped like a bottle brush, is referred to as a proteoglycan. Located primarily on the surface of cells, GAGs are characterized by high viscosity and low compressibility. That makes them ideal as a lubricating fluid in the joints. Moreover, their rigidity provides structural integrity to tissues.

In a recent study, one group of men with early hardening of the coronary arteries was given 200 milligrams of GAGs daily, while another group received no treatment. After 18 months, deposits on the lining of the vessels were 7.5 times thicker in the untreated group than in the GAG group—a significant difference. We don't know precisely how GAGs achieve this, but in addition to strengthening blood-vessel walls, they may reduce cholesterol levels and "thin" the blood, preventing its coagulation.

Other clinical studies have demonstrated that supplementing the diet with GAGs has a substantial effect on the structure, function, and integrity of arteries, easing the flow of blood. Improving cerebral (brain) and peripheral (in hands and feet) blood flow helps lessen the symptoms of cerebral vascular insufficiency—which can include short-term memory loss, vertigo, headache, ringing of the ears, and depression—and peripheral vascular disease—coldness of the hands and feet, pain, muscle cramps, and impotence.

Because of the effect GAGs have on blood-vessel walls, they are also essential in maintaining the structure and integrity of the veins. Without proper structural support, veins will lose their shape and become bulging and unsightly, causing such symptoms as a sense of heaviness in the legs, tingling sensations, fluid retention, itchiness, and painful cramps. Several researchers have, in fact, suggested that GAGs should be used as the "drug of first choice" in the nonsurgical treatment of varicose veins and hemorrhoids.

Despite these promising reviews, however, it's worth remembering that the therapeutic effects of GAGs still need to be confirmed by the type of large, double-blind trial in which neither the researchers nor the patients know who's getting the real drug.

Avoid if . . .

If you have a blood clotting disorder or liver or kidney disease, use GAGs only under a doctor's supervision.

Special Cautions

Even if GAGs seem to relieve your circulatory problem, it's essential to see a doctor about any type of cardiovascular disorder. Even phlebitis, for instance, is a potentially deadly disease.

Possible Drug Interactions

If you are taking drugs that reduce blood clotting—including Coumadin (warfarin sodium), heparin, Trental (pentoxifylline), and even aspirin—do not use GAGs except under a physician's supervision. Because GAGs tend to thin the blood, there is a chance that the combination could cause bleeding problems.

Special Information if You Are Pregnant or Breast-feeding

The safety of GAG supplements during pregnancy and breast-feeding has not been evaluated. Because they're taken only for their long-term benefits, the safest course is to forgo their use during this critical period.

Available Preparations and Dosage

The GAGs used in supplements are commercially produced from chondroitin sulfate, cartilage, bone, or the aortas (the largest artery) of cows. A typical dosage of aortic GAGs is 100 milligrams daily. Follow the supplier's directions. Take with meals to avoid any potential gastrointestinal upsets.

Overdosage
No information is available.

Grape Seed Extract

Why People Take It
Grape Seed Extract is used in the treatment of (peripheral venous insufficiency) poor circulation in the legs. In a study of more than 4,700 women with this condition, four out of five experienced improvement after taking 150 milligrams of this preparation twice a day for three months. Their legs felt lighter; did not burn, prickle, or tingle as much; and were less swollen and blue. The women also had fewer leg cramps at night.

What It Is; How It Works
Proanthocyanidins, a class of compounds found in grape seeds, strengthen the tiny blood vessels called capillaries, preventing leakage and reducing swelling in nearby tissues. They also help prevent unstable oxygen molecules called free radicals from getting out of control and doing

harm to the body. This antioxidant effect serves to reduce the oxidation of so-called bad cholesterol, thereby discouraging the buildup of the artery-clogging plaque that leads to stroke and heart attacks. The extract's antioxidant properties have also been found to limit the growth of tumors in laboratory animals.

There's at least some reason to believe that proanthocyanidins can also protect the liver from damage by the popular painkiller acetaminophen, improve vision in older adults, boost heart function, reduce swelling after surgery, and even promote hair growth. However, all of these possibilities await final verification.

Native to southern Europe and western Asia, grapevines are now grown in all temperate regions of the world. The leaves, fruit, and juice have all been used medicinally, but Grape Seed Extract produces the most pronounced therapeutic effects.

Avoid if . . .
No known medical condition precludes the use of Grape Seed Extract.

Special Cautions
Grape Seed Extract has no reported side effects.

Possible Drug Interactions
No interactions have been reported.

Special Information if You Are Pregnant or Breast-feeding
No harmful effects are known. As with all nutritional supplements, however, it's best to check with your doctor before taking it during this critical period.

Available Preparations and Dosage

Grape Seed Extract is available commercially in capsule and tablet form. Typical dosage recommendations for treatment of poor circulation range from 150 to 600 milligrams, taken in two or more smaller doses. For preventive therapy, daily doses of 50 milligrams are sometimes recommended.

Overdosage

Proanthocyanidins are water-soluble, so any excess intake is quickly eliminated in the urine.

Histidine

Why People Take It

Scientists know that this amino acid is important—lack of an adequate supply can stunt a youngster's growth—but they have yet to understand its full impact on the body. The only clinically tested therapeutic use of Histidine is in the treatment of rheumatoid arthritis, a disease that's sometimes accompanied by low levels of Histidine. However, the few trials conducted for this purpose were inconclusive, and little work has been done in the past 20 years.

Even Histidine's proponents make few other claims

for it. Some say it can remedy digestive problems by stimulating gastric secretions. Others claim it can enhance sexual pleasure by increasing circulation in the sex organs. However, no research has been done to confirm either of these effects.

What It Is; How It Works

Amino acids are the building blocks of human protein—a vital component in all of the body's cells. Histidine is one of several amino acids that the body can manufacture when dietary supplies fall short. For that reason it is considered "nonessential" in adults, who require only modest amounts. Growing children, on the other hand, need more than the body can produce, making it an essential part of a youngster's diet.

Histidine seems to play an important role in the production of histamine, a chemical that, among other things, stimulates digestion and dilates the arteries. Histidine also seems to be necessary for production of red and white blood cells, and may help support the activity of the immune system. It can bind and transport several metals, including copper and iron, and is said to be essential for zinc absorption. It plays a role in protecting the body from the effects of the sun, and may be helpful in maintaining the myelin sheaths that protect nerve cells. In children, a deficiency retards growth; in adults, a shortage is said to cause deafness.

Like all amino acids, Histidine is plentiful in high-protein foods such as eggs, meat, poultry, and fish.

Avoid if . . .

Some researchers have linked elevated levels of Histidine with anxiety and schizophrenia. If you have a history of mental illness, it's best to take Histidine only under a doctor's supervision.

Excess protein is either converted to energy or stored as fat, and because waste products from this conversion are eliminated in the urine, too much protein (or amino acid) intake can put a strain on the kidneys and liver. If you have kidney or liver disease, don't take any supplemental amino acids without your doctor's approval.

Special Cautions

Histidine supplements have no reported side effects.

Possible Drug Interactions

Histidine has not been well studied; no drug interactions are known.

Special Information if You Are Pregnant or Breast-feeding

There is no information on the effect of Histidine supplements during pregnancy. Since their safety during this critical period remains unverified, it's best to avoid them.

Available Preparations and Dosage

There is no official recommended dietary allowance for nonessential amino acids such as Histidine. Doses of between 1 and 8 grams a day have been used in clinical trials.

Histidine is available in tablet, capsule, and powder form, commonly in doses of 500 or 600 milligrams. It is also sold in combination with other amino acids.

Overdosage
No specific information on Histidine overdosage is available. However, even large doses of nonessential amino acids are unlikely to cause severe problems.

HMB
(Hydroxymethylbutyrate)

Why People Take It
This exotic bodybuilding aid is derived from the amino acid leucine, which itself is taken to enhance muscle bulk (see the entry on branched-chain amino acids). Although the evidence is still sketchy, HMB is said to improve strength and muscle mass, decrease fat, and reduce muscle damage and soreness for some individuals involved in weight-training programs.

What It Is; How It Works
Also known as beta-hydroxy beta-methylbutyrate (BHMB), HMB supplements were first developed for cattle feed by researchers at Iowa State University. But despite this less-than-glamorous past, HMB is rapidly gaining popularity as a dietary supplement for competitive athletes.

The rationale goes like this: Amino acids are the building blocks of human protein, and leucine in particular plays an essential role in growth. Along with the other branched-chain amino acids (isoleucine and valine), leucine is said to reduce protein breakdown in the muscles during periods of intense physical stress. Proponents of HMB hope that it, as a by-product of leucine metabolism, will provide similar benefits.

Although the research on HMB supplementation in humans is still considered preliminary, several recently published articles and abstracts support the theory that HMB can enhance the effects of vigorous exercise by building muscle and reducing body fat. In one study conducted at Iowa State University, 40 men received either HMB (3 grams per day) or a dummy supplement. All underwent four weeks of weight training, three times a week. At the end of the four weeks, the group taking the HMB showed more increase in muscle, less fat, and greater strength than those not taking HMB.

Because of studies like this, HMB is now being promoted as a safe alternative to anabolic steroids (which, while they build muscle, are both unsafe and illegal). However, other studies have detected no significant effects of HMB supplementation in well-trained athletes, so HMB's true value remains uncertain.

Avoid if . . .
If you have a medical problem, particularly with the liver or kidneys, check with your doctor before taking HMB.

Special Cautions
For use by healthy adults only. There are no reported side effects in short-term clinical studies, but researchers are still examining the supplement's long-term safety.

Remember that HMB is not a miracle pill. If it is capable of producing any benefits at all, you certainly won't see them unless you work out regularly.

Possible Drug Interactions
Some bodybuilders advocate "stacking"—that is, taking HMB with creatine. Thus far, there is no evidence that this is harmful (or helpful, for that matter).

Special Information if You Are Pregnant or Breast-feeding
The safety of HMB during pregnancy has not been evaluated. Since it's not needed to treat a disease, it should be avoided during pregnancy and breast-feeding.

Available Preparations and Dosage
Available in capsule or powder form, HMB is sometimes included in supplements with other performance-enhancing nutrients, such as creatine and protein. Proponents say that a dosage ranging from 1.5 to 4 grams per day can improve muscle size and strength.

You may want to start with 2 grams daily, taken with food. Many experts recommend limiting use of HMB to short intervals, up to three months—with three to four weeks off between cycles—until long-term studies confirm its safety.

Overdosage
No information on overdosage is available.

Inosine

Why People Take It

Inosine is one of the supplements that athletes take in the drive to boost performance. Closely related to the basic cellular "fuel" known as adenosine triphosphate (ATP), Inosine is said to increase energy, endurance, strength, and the body's ability to handle strenuous exercise and training. It is promoted to maintain and replenish levels of ATP, improve protein synthesis, speed recovery after exercise, and enhance the red blood cells' ability to carry oxygen to the muscles by increasing available levels of 2,3, diphosphoglycerate (2,3 DPG), a compound essential for the transport of oxygen.

Scientific research does not provide much support for these claims. Studies designed to confirm Inosine's ability to improve aerobic performance have produced mixed results. One study devoted specifically to 2,3, diphosphoglycerate levels has debunked the theory that Inosine supplements increase them. Studies of anaerobic performance (e.g., weight lifting) have not been conducted, and claims that Inosine is beneficial to muscle growth are based on speculation. On the other hand, some limited animal and human studies suggest that Inosine supplements may boost muscle function in the heart.

What It Is; How It Works
In theory, Inosine promotes the release of energy from ATP within the cells, thereby boosting the strength of muscular contractions, including those of the heart. In practice, it's unclear whether Inosine supplements make much of a difference.

Natural sources of Inosine include brewer's yeast and organ meats such as liver.

Avoid if . . .
Do not take an Inosine supplement if you have a disease affecting the kidneys.

Special Cautions
The body converts unused Inosine into uric acid. This could aggravate your condition if you have gout, a disease in which crystals of uric acid cause pain in the joints. No other side effects have been reported.

Possible Drug Interactions
No drug interactions are known.

Special Information if You Are Pregnant or Breast-feeding
Although there's no reason to expect harmful effects from Inosine, it has not been tested for safety during pregnancy and should therefore be avoided.

Available Preparations and Dosage

Inosine supplements come in tablet and powder forms, often as part of a multi-ingredient sports supplement. Powdered supplements are mixed with 8 to 12 ounces of water and taken prior to major workouts or competition.

There is no dietary requirement for Inosine and no official dosage recommendation. Some athletes take as much as 5 to 8 grams per day.

Overdosage

No information on overdosage is available.

Inositol

Why People Take It

Because Inositol seems to reduce high cholesterol levels, it can be used along with other treatments to help prevent clogged arteries and heart disease in people with unhealthy cholesterol levels. It may also prove helpful in reversing the peripheral neuropathy (tingling or numbness of hands and feet) that often accompanies diabetes. It has been used as a remedy for hair loss and eczema. And most recently it has been studied as a possible treatment for anxiety and mood disorders, including obsessive-compulsive disorder, depression, and panic disorder.

What It Is; How It Works

Inositol is naturally present in the cells of most plants and animals. In humans, it promotes the production of lecithin, a compound that aids in the transport of fat to the cells of the body and promotes its conversion to energy. It is by encouraging the proper use of fat that Inositol is thought to lower cholesterol.

Inositol is found in especially large concentrations in the brain and spine, where it may help support nerve transmission. Recent studies suggest that it may help regulate levels of the chemical messenger serotonin, accounting for its mood-altering effect. It also seems vital for healthy eyes, hair, bone marrow, and intestines.

A deficiency of Inositol is highly unlikely. It's manufactured by the body, and is part of the vitamin B complex in the foods that we eat. It is abundant in foods such as beans and lentils, liver, cantaloupe, citrus fruits other than lemons, nuts, oats, rice, wheat germ, and whole grains. Nutritionists estimate that the average daily consumption of Inositol ranges from 300 to 1,000 milligrams a day.

Avoid if . . .

Although Inositol is not known to have any toxic side effects, it's not recommended for healthy people, who ordinarily have an ample supply.

Special Cautions

If you are diabetic, have high cholesterol, or are considering using Inositol for a problem such as peripheral neuropathy or depression, be sure to check with your doctor before you begin. While Inositol may improve symptoms in some cases, it is not a cure for these conditions, and other types of treatment may be needed as well.

Possible Drug Interactions
No drug interactions are known.

Special Information if You Are Pregnant or Breast-feeding
There is no reason to believe that Inositol is harmful during pregnancy. Nevertheless, it's best to consult your doctor before taking any type of supplement at this critical time.

Available Preparations and Dosage
Inositol, either synthetic or natural, is available as capsules and powder, and is also often part of lecithin supplements. There is no official recommended dietary allowance (RDA) for Inositol, but doctors typically suggest 500 to 1,000 milligrams daily. Some multivitamin tablets contain Inositol, but in amounts too small to be of any significance.

Overdosage
High doses of Inositol seem free of problems, but no specific information on overdosage is available.

Ipriflavone

Why People Take It

A synthetic form of plant-based estrogen, Ipriflavone has drawn interest primarily because of its beneficial action against postmenopausal bone loss. Researchers hope that it may help prevent osteoporosis without incurring the risks associated with regular estrogen, the treatment against which all other bone-saving drugs are compared.

After many decades of use, estrogen is known to prevent bone loss and help build thicker bones—effects that reduce the chance of fractures. It also relieves symptoms of menopause and provides some protection against heart disease. However, estrogen can increase the risk of cancers of the breast and uterus. Progesterone, another hormone, is prescribed with estrogen to reduce the threat of uterine tumors, but its use does not protect breast tissue. Not surprisingly, researchers continue to look for a safer alternative that is equally effective in preventing and treating osteoporosis, if not in other areas as well.

Research suggests that Ipriflavone may indeed be able to play such a role. Studies have confirmed that it does slow bone loss, although whether or not it increases bone density to any significant degree remains to be seen. Some data also suggest that Ipriflavone may fortify the effects of low doses of estrogen, helping to produce a greater effect on bones. On the downside, though, Ipriflavone also seems to increase estrogen's effect on the uterus, so that combining the two may be too risky for some women. Other studies have shown that Ipriflavone might be useful in the treatment of Paget's disease of bone, a painful bone-deforming ailment. In clinical trials, it reduced the aching discomfort that plagues people with this illness.

Some advocates say that Ipriflavone is a useful tool for bodybuilders, suggesting that it can help produce lean muscle. Scientists generally dismiss this claim, concentrating on its potential for slowing bone loss. Ipriflavone is sold as an osteoporosis remedy in Italy, Japan, and the United Kingdom, but remains an experimental drug in the United States, where more rigorous tests are required. For example, researchers will want to see how Ipriflavone stacks up against other osteoporosis treatments and whether its beneficial effect on bone actually results in a lower risk of fractures.

What It Is; How It Works

Ipriflavone is modeled after a compound called daidzein, found naturally in soybeans. Daidzein is a member of a group of beneficial nutrients called soy isoflavones (see separate entry) that may possess cancer-fighting properties. Due to its estrogenlike effect on bone, it is also classified as a phytoestrogen (*phyto* for "plant"). (See separate entry.)

Nobody knows why Ipriflavone seems to stall bone

loss. Bones undergo constant renewal through the cooperative efforts of two types of cells: osteoblasts, which make new bone, and osteoclasts, which clear away old bone. After age 30, the osteoclasts begin to get rid of old bone faster than the osteoblasts can produce new material, a situation that worsens after menopause. Some researchers suggest that Ipriflavone may stunt the activity or development of the destructive osteoclasts. Others theorize that it may promote the activity or development of the nurturing osteoblasts. A third hypothesis holds that Ipriflavone spurs the body to release calcitonin, a hormone that prevents bone loss by diminishing the number of osteoclasts and their ability to function. (In nasal spray or injection form, calcitonin is frequently used in the treatment of osteoporosis.)

Avoid if . . .
Never use Ipriflavone while taking estrogen, since it could increase the hormone's negative effects. Also avoid Ipriflavone if you've ever had an allergic reaction to it.

Special Cautions
If you have kidney disease, take Ipriflavone only under a doctor's supervision; you could build up excessive levels of the drug. In fact, anyone with kidney disease should check with her doctor about taking smaller amounts of Ipriflavone than generally advised on the label.

Ipriflavone appears to have few side effects. The most common complaints are stomach pain or burning and diarrhea.

Possible Drug Interactions

Ipriflavone impairs the body's ability to eliminate the asthma drug theophylline, and can produce elevated blood levels of the drug, almost as if higher doses were suddenly being taken. As a result, people who combine Ipriflavone and theophylline could develop symptoms of theophylline toxicity, such as nausea, vomiting, a racing heartbeat, or seizures. Researchers think Ipriflavone may interact with other important drugs as well, including phenytoin, an anticonvulsant; warfarin, a blood thinner; and tolbutamide, which is used to treat people with diabetes. Given Ipriflavone's interaction potential, it's wise to check with your doctor before combining it with any other medication.

Special Information if You Are Pregnant or Breast-feeding

Regular estrogen must never be taken during pregnancy, since it can cause the developing baby significant harm. It's not known whether plant-based estrogens pose a similar danger. However, since Ipriflavone is considered useful only for *postmenopausal* bone loss, there's no valid reason for taking it during pregnancy in any event.

Available Preparations and Dosage

Ipriflavone is taken by mouth and may be sold alone or in combination with calcium and other vitamins or minerals. The usual dosage is 600 milligrams of Ipriflavone per day. How many times per day you take the drug depends on the contents of the pills that you've purchased. For example, a pill containing 300 milligrams of Ipriflavone would be taken twice a day, while one containing 200 milligrams would be taken three times a day.

Overdosage
No information on overdosage is available.

Lactobacillus

Why People Take It
The human digestive tract is inhabited by a variety of beneficial bacteria referred to as probiotics. Among the most important of these friendly fellow travelers are the Lactobacillus species, especially *Lactobacillus acidophilus* (probably best known for its role in reestablishing friendly bacteria in the colon after a course of antibiotics), *Lactobacillus bifidis* (more common in babies), and *Lactobacillus GG*, a newly identified type of Lactobacillus particularly useful for postantibiotic bouts of diarrhea.

What It Is; How It Works
The Lactobacillus group helps to maintain a healthy environment in the intestines by producing lactic acid, acetic acid, hydrogen peroxide, and other organic compounds that increase acidity inside the intestine and discourage the reproduction of many harmful bacteria. Lactobacillus species also produce bacteriocins, natural antibiotics that kill a variety of detrimental organisms.

The anti-infective properties of these probiotic bacteria make them potentially helpful in the prevention of recurrent vaginal yeast infections. Lactobacillus supplements can also reduce your chances of getting traveler's diarrhea and may prevent renewed attacks. Reports also suggest a beneficial impact on stomach and digestive upset, indigestion and heartburn, intestinal gas, irritable bowel syndrome, and gastrointestinal inflammation.

Lactobacillus acidophilus is the most common probiotic supplement. It's taken to restore intestinal balance after bouts of diarrhea, and to maintain general intestinal health. As a source of lactase (the enzyme needed for the digestion of milk), it may also help relieve lactose intolerance, although conclusive proof of this is lacking. Other largely unverified claims for acidophilus assert that it improves immunity, helps allergies, improves skin, relieves canker sores, reduces cholesterol levels, alleviates constipation, improves acne, and lessens the risk of colon cancer.

Lactobacillus bifidis performs essentially the same functions as acidophilus, but is more prevalent in the digestive tracts of infants and may be more protective against such food-borne infections as salmonellosis.

Lactobacillus GG, one of the newest of the probiotics, has recently sparked considerable excitement as a remedy for antibiotic-induced diarrhea, digestive problems, and vaginal yeast infections. Antibiotics prescribed to kill harmful bacteria frequently kill the beneficial ones as well. *Lactobacillus GG* seems to be particularly good at reestablishing friendly intestinal organisms, possibly because it survives stomach acids better than acidophilus. In any event, clinical research has shown it to significantly cut the rate of antibiotic-induced diarrhea, as well as many other types of the disorder.

Lactobacillus supplements are totally unnecessary as long as your native population of probiotic bacteria maintain their health. However, antibiotics, chronic diarrhea, and poor eating habits often serve to give harmful bacteria the upper hand, while emotional stress seems to lower the count of friendly ones. If you face any one of these problems, extra probiotics might prove beneficial.

Avoid if . . .
There's no known reason to avoid probiotics.

Special Cautions
The safety of Lactobacillus is well documented. It has been used since the early 1900s in the fermentation of products such as yogurt, buttermilk, cheese, and sourdough. In fact, acidophilus milk and many yogurt products contain live bacteria and are sometimes used to maintain intestinal health, though the bacteria count in these products is not very high.

Because Lactobacillus supplements contain living organisms, freshness is important. Purchase products containing lactobacilli well before their expiration date. Refrigerate the supplements once you have opened them, and throw them out when they are more than six months old. At that point, the organisms are dead.

Possible Drug Interactions
Although Lactobacillus supplements can often remedy antibiotic-induced diarrhea, they do not interfere with the therapeutic action of the antibiotic itself.

Special Information if You Are Pregnant or Breast-feeding
No specific information is available. However, it's wise to check with your doctor before taking any supplement while pregnant or breast-feeding.

Available Preparations and Dosage
Lactobacillus supplements are available as powders, capsules, tablets, and liquids. The count of live bacteria in these products is in the millions and billions per daily dose. Generally, 1 to 2 billion colony forming units (CFUs) of acidophilus per day is considered sufficient to keep intestinal probiotic bacteria in tip-top shape. Larger doses may be warranted if the population is depleted.

Most experts advise against taking Lactobacillus supplements continuously. Instead, they recommend reserving them for short courses to repopulate the colon with friendly flora after antibiotic therapy, to treat intestinal yeast overgrowth, or to stave off infectious diarrhea when traveling in underdeveloped countries.

Overdosage
Even large doses of Lactobacillus have no reported side effects.

Lecithin

Why People Take It

Commercial Lecithin supplements are composed primarily of choline and inositol, two fatty compounds that help support the integrity of the body's cell membranes while aiding the transport of fats into the cells and regulating cholesterol levels. (See separate entries.) Lecithin supplements can produce a significant reduction in cholesterol levels, which in turn may stave off the buildup of artery-clogging plaque and help prevent heart disease.

Because choline and inositol have been associated with the regulation of various chemical messengers in the nervous system, they've also been proposed as treatments for Alzheimer's disease and several neurological disorders. Studies to date, however, have revealed little if any benefit in such cases. The primary value of Lecithin supplements remains in their effect on cholesterol.

What It Is; How It Works

Discussions of Lecithin can be confusing, since scientists use the term as a synonym for phosphatidylcholine, one of the ingredients of commercial Lecithin supplements. Phosphatidylcholine by itself can be taken to fight high cholesterol (see separate entry). The phosphatidylcholine content of commercial Lecithin products ranges from 5 to 30 percent.

In addition to lowering cholesterol, the phosphatidyl-choline in Lecithin products may fight heart disease by acting as a blood thinner, discouraging the clumping of blood platelets that can sometimes produce dangerous clotting in the bloodstream. The choline found in phosphatidylcholine also supports the health of the liver and may be helpful in preventing or treating liver disorders such as cirrhosis, fatty liver, hepatitis, and damage from toxic substances.

The richest dietary sources of Lecithin are egg yolks and organ meats such as liver. Since these foods are also high in cholesterol and saturated fats, some nutritionists fear that the current drive for low-cholesterol diets could be leading to deficiencies of Lecithin and choline in some people. If you're concerned about this, soybean products and vegetables such as cabbage and cauliflower will provide you with good alternative sources of choline. Lecithin is also found in a number of processed foods, where it is used as an emulsifier to keep oil and water from separating and to retard spoilage.

Avoid if . . .

Pure choline supplements are not recommended for people with ulcers, bipolar disorder, or Parkinson's disease. Although commercial Lecithin supplements are less potent, you still may want to avoid them under these circumstances.

Special Cautions

Potential side effects include nausea, upset stomach, abdominal discomfort, diarrhea, and stiff muscles. The likelihood of side effects increases with the size of the dose.

If you're on a low-fat diet, be aware that regular doses of Lecithin will significantly boost your fat intake.

Possible Drug Interactions

Because the choline in Lecithin supplements can boost levels of the chemical messenger acetylcholine, you should avoid combining these supplements with a prescription drug such as scopolamine (an antinausea medication) that works by blocking the effects of acetylcholine.

Special Information if You Are Pregnant or Breast-feeding

There is no reason to believe that ordinary amounts of Lecithin are harmful during pregnancy. Nevertheless, it's best to consult your doctor before taking any type of supplement at this critical time.

Available Preparations and Dosage

Lecithin is available in liquid, powder, granule, and capsule form. Dosage recommendations vary with the amount of choline in the supplement. For a medium-potency product, doses can range from 5 to 10 grams daily. Follow the manufacturer's directions, and to benefit from Lecithin's ability to help break down fats, take it just prior to, or with, meals.

Overdosage

No information on overdosage is available.

Lipoic Acid

Why People Take It

A vitaminlike substance with antioxidant properties, Lipoic Acid also acts as a cofactor in the conversion of blood sugar (glucose) into energy. In Germany it's an approved treatment for a painful degenerative nerve condition called diabetic neuropathy, as well as other complications of diabetes. (Diabetic neuropathy is thought to be caused in part by oxidative stress.) Lipoic Acid is also used in Europe as a treatment for mushroom poisoning.

Laboratory research on Lipoic Acid suggests other potential benefits. Several studies on animals have found that it improves their memory and cognitive function, prevents cataract formation, and lowers their blood pressure. Possibly because of its antioxidant effect, it has also shown promise for certain kidney and liver conditions. At this point, however, we don't know whether it has the same effects in humans.

Manufacturers of Lipoic Acid recommend it as a treatment for AIDS, on the basis of a study in which it prevented the reproduction of the HIV virus in test tubes. Promoters also claim that it can improve muscle performance, slow the aging process, remedy glaucoma and many other conditions, and protect against liver disease, heart disease, and cancer. Unfortunately, most of these claims are based either on animal studies or the known antioxidant action of Lipoic Acid, and there is currently no proof that it has the same effects on humans.

What It Is; How It Works

Lipoic Acid is manufactured by the body, so deficiencies are unknown and it's not classified as a dietary essential. It can, however, be obtained from red meats, liver, and yeast. It is sometimes called the perfect antioxidant because it is both fat- and water-soluble.

In its role as an antioxidant, Lipoic Acid acts as a free-radical scavenger. Free radicals are highly reactive unpaired molecules that cruise the bloodstream looking for other unpaired molecules to combine with. If they link up with the wrong molecules in healthy cells, oxidation and damage result. While free radicals are products of the normal metabolic process, environmental pollution, smoking, the effects of the sun, and a poor diet can foster excessive amounts. Lipoic Acid not only neutralizes free radicals itself, but also seems to help recycle other antioxidant agents with similar abilities, such as vitamins C and E, as well as glutathione.

Avoid if . . .

No known medical conditions preclude the use of Lipoic Acid.

Special Cautions

If you take Lipoic Acid for diabetes, remember that it's not a substitute for other forms of treatment. Continue to follow the plan your doctor recommends and carefully monitor your blood sugar. Similarly, you can't rely on Lipoic Acid as a replacement for prescription HIV drugs.

Possible Drug Interactions
Diabetics may have to readjust their insulin intake when taking high doses of Lipoic Acid. If you feel light-headed after taking this supplement, check your blood sugar and adjust your insulin according to your doctor's instructions.

Special Information if You Are Pregnant or Breast-feeding
Although Lipoic Acid is a natural bodily substance, the effects of high doses during pregnancy are unknown. As with all nutritional supplements, it's best to check with your doctor before taking it during these critical periods.

Available Preparations and Dosage
It is available as a nutritional supplement in 50- to 200-milligram capsules. Manufacturers recommend taking 50 milligrams per day as an antioxidant, 300 to 600 milligrams per day for diabetes-related conditions, and 150 milligrams three times daily for AIDS.

Overdosage
There are no reports of overdosage with Lipoic Acid.

Lutein

Why People Take It

Lutein offers powerful protection against two serious eye problems. It significantly reduces the odds of developing macular degeneration, a wasting of the retina that leads to irreversible blindness in many older adults. It's also one of the nutrients thought to protect against cataracts, cloudy areas on the lens of the eye that eventually afflict more than half of all senior Americans.

Lutein may also be one of the key elements that lend certain vegetables their ability to fend off colon cancer. And ongoing research is investigating Lutein's role in protecting the skin from sun damage, as well as its potentially heart-healthy effects on cholesterol.

What It Is; How It Works

Lutein is one of the carotenoids, a large group of antioxidants that protect the body's cells from the harmful molecules called free radicals. A light-absorbing pigment related to vitamin A, Lutein is not produced by the body and so must be obtained from food or vitamin supplements. It is one of two pigments that seem to filter damaging forms of light from reaching the macula, or central region of the retina. The macula is responsible for straight-ahead vision and visual sharpness. It can eventually succumb to damage from free radicals, poor circulation, and overexposure to UV sun rays. Currently, 90 percent of the people with macular degeneration fail to respond to treatment, so prevention remains crucial. Those most at risk for macular degeneration are smokers and people with light-colored eyes.

A study conducted in 1994 showed that people with the highest intakes of six carotenoids, including Lutein, and three vitamins (A, C, and E) enjoyed 43 percent less risk of macular degeneration than those with the lowest intakes. And those who ate a diet rich specifically in Lutein and zeaxanthin, another carotenoid, had a 57 percent reduction in risk. Likewise, diets high in Lutein seem to be associated with a lower risk of cataracts, possibly by protecting the lens from light-induced free radicals.

Lutein's reputation as a potential cancer-fighter rests on a recent study that concluded that, of all the many carotenoids that occur in vegetables, Lutein demonstrates the strongest protective effects against colon cancer. (It was also found to improve chances of recovery in certain cases.) Lutein may also discourage the development of skin cancer by protecting the skin from damaging UVA rays.

Avoid if . . .
There are no known reasons to avoid Lutein supplements.

Special Cautions
No side effects have been reported.

Possible Drug Interactions
No interactions are known.

Special Information if You Are Pregnant or Breast-feeding
There's no reason to expect any harm from Lutein. However, it's wise to check with your doctor before taking any supplement while pregnant or breast-feeding.

Available Preparations and Dosage
The best dietary sources of Lutein include spinach, collard greens, kale, mustard greens, turnip greens, romaine lettuce, peas, and leeks. It is also included in a number of multivitamin formulas and eye care supplements, and can be purchased as an individual supplement in capsule, softgel (gel cap), or tablet form.

In studies of macular degeneration, intake of about 6 milligrams of Lutein per day has shown a protective effect. A large bowl of spinach salad will provide the necessary amount. If you choose to take a Lutein supplement, combine it with the related carotenoid zeaxanthin, and take it with food to improve absorption.

Overdosage
No information on overdosage is available.

Lycopene

Why People Take It

Lycopene, a compound found in fruits and vegetables (especially tomatoes), has been associated with a reduced risk of heart attack. It is also thought to provide a certain amount of protection against some types of cancer, particularly cancers of the prostate or breast.

Most evidence of Lycopene's benefit comes from studies comparing disease rates in groups of people with diets high or low in Lycopene-rich foods. Such foods contain other substances, such as beta-carotene and fiber, that may have contributed to the effects the researchers observed. Still, that hasn't stopped vitamin manufacturers from rolling out tomato-oil capsules and other supplements containing Lycopene alone.

Although these products may well confer benefits similar to those of a Lycopene-rich diet, that has yet to be confirmed by large-scale testing. As long as the jury remains out, most experts recommend enjoying more red sauce and ketchup instead of popping Lycopene pills.

What It Is; How it Works

Lycopene is one of the carotenoids, a group of naturally occurring plant chemicals found in yellow, orange, red, and leafy green vegetables and fruits. Researchers have established that Lycopene, the most common carotenoid in the American diet and the human body, is a powerful antioxidant. Oxidation is a chemical process (akin to burning) that produces toxic compounds called free radicals. These compounds react easily with surrounding tissues, triggering a host of damaging effects, from aging to cancer development. Lycopene scavenges free radicals in the body, guarding various types of cells (including immune cells) against their attack.

True to its antioxidant nature, Lycopene has been shown to suppress the growth of cancer cells in laboratory and animal studies. And recent studies in humans have bolstered these findings, showing significant benefits from elevated Lycopene levels both in the diet and in the body.

- In a study of more than 47,000 men, those who ate tomato products at least 10 times a week had less than half the risk of developing advanced prostate cancer compared to men who ate such products less often.
- A review of 72 studies of the cancer prevention–tomato connection found that tomato intake was linked to reduced risk in 57 studies, with the connection considered statistically reliable in 35. (The studies, however, were analyses of disease rates in various groups, rather than actual clinical trials.)
- Prostate cancer patients have been shown to have lower Lycopene levels in their prostate tissue and blood

than those found in healthy men; this relationship is
more pronounced for Lycopene than for any other
carotenoid.

• In a small study of 33 men facing prostate surgery,
those who took Lycopene supplements for 30 days before the operation were less likely to have their cancer
spread than those who took no supplements.

• In a multicenter European study, higher levels of carotenoids in fatty tissue were associated with a lower
risk for heart attack.

The richest and best-absorbed sources of Lycopene are
cooked tomato products such as tomato sauce and paste
or tomato ketchup. Lycopene is also present in watermelon, tomato juice, raw tomatoes, and pink grapefruit.

Why not just swallow a Lycopene pill? The benefits of
taking this compound in isolation from its chemical fellow
travelers are still uncertain. Lycopene supplements lack
many of the complex substances found in fresh or cooked
fruits and vegetables, including dietary fiber, vitamins,
minerals, and other phytochemicals (plant chemicals)—
substances that may turn out to be responsible for at least
some of the beneficial impact of Lycopene-rich foods.
Carotenoids may also interact with one another, and it's
unknown whether supplementing one carotenoid might
impair the absorption of others.

Avoid if . . .
The effects of habitual, long-term Lycopene supplementation, and its potential for toxicity, are still unknown. At
this point, however, there appear to be no well-established
medical reasons to avoid Lycopene.

Special Cautions

Concerns have been raised as to whether Lycopene may skew the results of testing for prostate-specific antigen (PSA), a substance in the blood that signals the possibility of prostate cancer. If you're taking Lycopene, be sure to tell the doctor before undergoing a PSA test.

Possible Drug Interactions

There are no well-known drug interactions for Lycopene. However, tell your doctor if you are taking this or other supplements before starting any new medication.

Special Information if You Are Pregnant or Breast-feeding

The effect of large doses of Lycopene on a developing baby remain unknown. Since the supplement isn't necessary for your short-term health, it's best to avoid it during pregnancy and nursing. Stick to dietary sources of the compound, which are high in other vital nutrients as well.

Available Preparations and Dosage

There is no officially recommended dietary allowance for Lycopene, and researchers have yet to establish an optimal dosage for cancer prevention and other health benefits. In one study, the men with the lowest rate of cancer had at least 6.5 milligrams of Lycopene in their diets a day—approximately the amount in one cup of cubed watermelon, two medium tomatoes, or half a cup of tomato sauce.

If you choose to take a pill, supplements containing from 3 to 15 milligrams of Lycopene are available.

Overdosage

Doctors don't yet know whether a high dose of Lycopene could prove harmful, or what the size of such a dose would be. However, it's wise not to exceed the dosage recommended by a supplement's manufacturer.

Lysine

Why People Take It

Although Lysine has been part of everyone's diet since the dawn of mankind, medical researchers have only recently identified two properties that suggest it could be a useful medication. Some studies have found that it can block proliferation of the herpes simplex virus, raising the possibility of using it as a remedy for cold sores and genital herpes. Other research has revealed that it plays an important role in the absorption and conservation of calcium, making it a potential weapon in the battle against osteoporosis. Although neither benefit has been confirmed conclusively, experts say the results of the studies to date are promising, and more research should be done.

Some proponents insist that Lysine also maintains healthy blood vessels and helps build muscle, but these claims have yet to be verified.

What It Is; How It Works

Lysine is one of the eight amino acids deemed essential
in the diet, since the body is unable to manufacture its
own supply. It's a vital component of numerous proteins
needed to build and repair tissue and synthesize adequate
supplies of hormones, enzymes, and antibodies. In addition to its role in conserving calcium, it helps form the
collagen that makes up cartilage and connective tissues.

Poultry, eggs, fish, dairy products, meat, beans, yeast,
and nuts all provide abundant amounts of Lysine, so deficiencies of this nutrient are virtually unknown in the
United States. Even strict vegetarians have enough in
their diet. Experts say the only possible exceptions might
be burn victims and strict vegetarians who are pregnant
or breast-feeding.

Avoid if . . .

High doses of amino acids lay an extra burden on the
liver and kidneys. If you have a problem in either area,
don't take Lysine without your doctor's approval. Also
avoid it if you have diabetes or an allergy to proteins
such as those found in eggs, milk, or wheat.

Special Cautions

In animal studies, Lysine has retarded growth in the
young. Lysine *supplements* are therefore not recommended for children. (Normal dietary levels of Lysine are
not a concern.)

Possible Drug Interactions

No drug interactions are known.

Special Information if You Are Pregnant or Breast-feeding
It's not known whether high doses of Lysine are safe
during pregnancy. As with any supplement not absolutely
necessary for your health, it's best to avoid using Lysine
while pregnant or breast-feeding.

Available Preparations and Dosage
Both natural and synthetic forms of Lysine are available, in
tablet and capsule form, most commonly in 500-milligram
strengths. Lysine is also included in many multivitamin
formulations.

Adults need a daily intake of approximately 5.5 milligrams of Lysine per pound of body weight. When Lysine
is taken for a herpes simplex infection, a typical dosage is
1,000 to 3,000 milligrams daily.

Overdosage
Unless you have an underlying disease, even high doses
of amino acids rarely cause problems. Sustained use of
excessive amounts of Lysine could, however, increase
your risk of gallstones, high cholesterol, or diarrhea.

Malate

Why People Take It

Supplement suppliers claim that Malate can improve the body's ability to absorb minerals. In the form of malic acid, it is often included in magnesium supplements that claim to relieve the nagging muscle aches of fibromyalgia. It's also taken by some athletes in hopes that it will boost their energy levels.

To date, there's no evidence that Malate can help achieve either of these goals. One animal study, published in 1986, hints that Malate supplements may increase the processing of certain chemicals in the body, but no human trials have verified an actual increase in energy. There are also no scientific studies confirming Malate's ability to relieve fibromyalgia.

What It Is; How It Works

Malate is produced by the body as it breaks apart the chemical bonds in carbohydrates, proteins, and fats in order to release their energy (a process called the Krebs cycle). When you are involved in endurance training, the amount of malate in your system increases as the Krebs cycle works to supply extra energy. It's this fact that leads some athletes to take Malate—and other by-products of the Krebs cycle—in an attempt to maximize the release of energy.

In the form of malic acid, Malate is found in a variety of foods, including apples and grapes. In fact, it's sometimes labeled "apple acid." It is used commercially in the aging of wine and as a food additive for flavoring of nonalcoholic beverages, chewing gum, hard candy, fruit juices, jams, and jellies.

Malate is also an ingredient in a number of prescription drugs, including medications for high blood pressure. It is often found in calcium supplements as well. For instance, calcium citrate–malate, which combines calcium with citric acid and malic acid, is considered by some to be the most easily absorbed calcium supplement.

Avoid if . . .
No known medical conditions preclude the use of malate.

Special Cautions
The Food and Drug Administration generally recognizes malic acid as safe when used as a food additive. However, its safety when used as a dietary supplement remains unknown. A number of Malate-containing supplements have in fact caused adverse effects. But since these supplements include ten or more substances, it's unclear which ingredient or combination of ingredients caused the adverse reaction.

Possible Drug Interactions
Check with your doctor before taking a Malate supplement if you are taking a medication that contains Malate or malic acid.

Special Information if You Are Pregnant or Breast-feeding
No harmful effects are known, but during this period it's
best to avoid taking any supplement that isn't mandatory for your health.

Available Preparations and Dosage
Malate supplements are available in tablet, capsule,
and powder forms. There is no official recommended dietary allowance, and manufacturers' dosage recommendations vary.

Overdosage
No information on overdosage is available.

Melatonin

Why People Take It
With its ability to regulate body rhythms and promote
normal sleep, this natural hormone has become a popular
alternative to artificial sleep aids. For many people, it
seems to relieve not only insomnia but jet lag and seasonal affective disorder (SAD) as well.

Other roles proposed for Melatonin are more controversial. Some advocates claim it can hold back the spread
of cancer. Others say it can delay the onset of aging,

combat the symptoms of Alzheimer's disease, lower cholesterol levels, and reduce high blood pressure. However, most doctors feel that its effectiveness for these purposes remains unproven.

What It Is; How It Works

Melatonin is a product of the pineal gland, where it is synthesized from the amino acid tryptophan. Under normal conditions, Melatonin levels foreshadow the sleep cycle, usually increasing rapidly from the late evening until midnight, then decreasing as morning approaches. In this way, Melatonin helps regulate circadian rhythm, the body's 24-hour "dark-light clock" that governs the timing of hormone production, sleep, body temperature, and more.

Not surprisingly, people with high levels of Melatonin usually sleep longer and more soundly than those with a deficiency. For example, the elderly, who produce less Melatonin than the young and middle-aged, are typically more susceptible to insomnia. Similarly, events that throw Melatonin levels out of synch, such as a jet trip between time zones, seem to interfere with production of the hormone and thus disrupt sleep. Consumption of alcohol, tobacco, and narcotics has a similar effect.

Some researchers speculate that chronically low Melatonin levels may also be linked with cancer, especially in the breast, skin, or prostate gland. They note that many cancer patients have poorly functioning pineal glands and show low levels of Melatonin. Boosting these levels, they theorize, might strengthen the immune system and stimulate it to kill malignant cells, or at least prevent the cells from dividing rapidly. Until further proof is available, however, Melatonin can be considered at best an adjunct to conventional treatment—and certainly not a substitute for it.

Avoid if . . .

Unless your doctor approves, do not take Melatonin if you have an autoimmune disease such as rheumatoid arthritis, any condition that affects your lymphatic system, AIDS, osteoarthritis, depression or any other emotional disorder, diabetes, epilepsy, heart disease, leukemia, multiple sclerosis, or serious allergies.

Couples who are trying to conceive a baby should avoid this hormone. It is also not for use by children or teenagers.

Special Cautions

Take Melatonin only at bedtime. Do not drive or operate machinery after taking a dose.

If you develop a headache, rash, or upset stomach, or find that your normal sleeping patterns are disrupted, stop taking Melatonin and check with your doctor.

Possible Drug Interactions

Check with your doctor before combining Melatonin with the following:

Beta-blockers such as Inderal, Lopressor, and
   Tenormin
Large amounts of ibuprofen (Motrin, Advil)
Mood-altering drugs such as diazepam (Valium)
Steroid medications such as prednisone

Special Information if You Are Pregnant or Breast-feeding
Do not take Melatonin supplements during pregnancy or while breast-feeding.

Available Preparations and Dosage
Melatonin is available without prescription in tablet and capsule form. Most experts recommend taking from 1 to 3 milligrams approximately 20 minutes before bedtime. Controlled-release formulations should be taken 2 hours before going to bed.

To determine the exact dosage that is best for you, ask your doctor to monitor your blood level and adjust the dosage accordingly. Do not attempt to medicate yourself.

Overdosage
Several physicians and researchers say that dosages as high as 200 milligrams of Melatonin per day appear to do no harm.

Methionine

Why People Take It
This sulfur-containing amino acid is one of several "lipotropic" substances that promote the processing of fats within the body. (Others are choline, inositol, and

lecithin. See separate entries.) In particular, Methionine helps clear fat out of the liver, and is used to treat certain types of liver damage.

Methionine also helps rid the body of toxins such as lead, mercury, and cadmium. This property has prompted some experts to speculate that Methionine could prove helpful in the treatment of such problems as depression, schizophrenia, Alzheimer's disease, other forms of dementia, hyperactivity in children, and kidney damage. There's currently little evidence to support these theories, although a Methionine-containing compound called SAMe has shown promise in the treatment of depression, osteoarthritis, and the muscle pain of fibromyalgia. (See separate entry.)

What It Is; How It Works

Methionine is one of the "essential" amino acids that can't be manufactured by the body and must be obtained from the diet. Like all amino acids, it's one of the raw materials the body uses to manufacture human proteins. Its sulfur content makes it especially important for the maintenance of healthy skin, hair, and nails, all of which are high in sulfur-containing keratin.

Methionine is required for the production of glutathionine, one of the body's chief natural detoxifiers (see separate entry). When higher levels of toxic compounds are present, more Methionine is needed. Abundant supplies are available in meat, fish, eggs, and dairy products, so supplementary Methionine is rarely needed by anyone other than a strict vegetarian.

Avoid if . . .

High doses of amino acids lay an extra burden on the liver and kidneys. If you have a problem in either area, don't take Methionine without your doctor's approval. Also avoid it if you have diabetes (which puts further stress on the kidneys) or an allergy to proteins such as those found in eggs, milk, or wheat.

Special Cautions

When taking a Methionine supplement, you might want to take a multivitamin as well. Excessive Methionine intake accompanied by a shortage of folic acid, vitamin B_6, and vitamin B_{12} can boost levels of homocysteine, a substance linked to heart disease and stroke.

Possible Drug Interactions

No drug interactions are known.

Special Information if You Are Pregnant or Breast-feeding

It's not known whether high doses of Methionine are safe during pregnancy. As with any supplement not absolutely necessary for your health, it's best to avoid using Methionine while pregnant or breast-feeding.

Available Preparations and Dosage

The average adult requires about 800 to 1,000 milligrams of Methionine per day, an amount exceeded by most Western diets. If you take Methionine for a liver ailment or a problem such as depression, proponents recommend taking anywhere from 200 to 400 milligrams two to three times a day. Methionine supplements are most often found in capsule form.

Overdosage

Unless you have an underlying disease, even high doses of amino acids rarely cause problems.

MSM (Methyl Sulfonyl Methane)

Why People Take It

According to its proponents, MSM relieves osteoarthritis pain. And because MSM is inexpensive and low in toxicity, people who haven't had good results with other treatments are often tempted to give it a try. Before you begin taking it, though, you should know that there's little carefully controlled research to back up its efficacy, and that individual experiments often prove nothing. As the Arthritis Foundation points out, symptoms of arthritis often come and go on their own, so any improvement could be a coincidence, particularly since MSM is said to take several weeks to produce its results.

What It Is; How It Works

MSM is an organic sulfur compound found naturally in the body. It is readily available in the diet through fresh fruits and vegetables, grains, fish, and milk. (Packaged foods may lack MSM, which breaks down during food processing.) The sulfur in MSM plays a variety of roles in the body. It's important for the maintenance of healthy skin, hair, and nails. More important, it appears to be necessary for the production of collagen, one of the major building blocks of the cartilage that cushions the joints.

MSM is chemically related to DMSO, a drug that enjoyed popularity in the 1960s as a purported antioxidant, anti-inflammatory, and antiarthritis agent. Despite these claims, DMSO has been judged effective by the FDA for only one ailment, a bladder inflammation called interstitial nephritis.

Advocates believe that MSM and DMSO share a similar mechanism of action. They think that both may slow transmission of pain impulses by the nerves, and perhaps help make the body's own inflammation fighter, cortisol, work more effectively. They claim that, in addition to osteoarthritis, MSM can relieve rheumatoid arthritis, fibromyalgia, gout, and chronic headache, as well as back pain.

There are a few unpublished studies on the claims for MSM, conducted by proponents, which seem to show that the product has helped people with osteoarthritis pain. These studies are impossible for experts to evaluate. They say MSM is worthy of further research, but at this point the work remains to be done.

Avoid if . . .
If you are healthy, you don't need supplemental MSM.

Special Cautions
If you have osteoarthritis, it's best to check with your doctor before starting MSM. There may be a more promising

alternative to try first. Remember, too, that the long-term effects of MSM are still unknown.

Possible Drug Interactions
Don't combine MSM with drugs that thin the blood, such as Coumadin or aspirin, since MSM may have a blood-thinning effect.

Special Information if You Are Pregnant or Breast-feeding
The effects of MSM in pregnancy are unknown. Avoid using it while pregnant or breast-feeding.

Available Preparations and Dosage
MSM is a white, odorless, slightly bitter powder which is easily dissolved. Proponents often recommend a starting dose of 1,000 milligrams daily, with up to 8,000 milligrams daily considered safe. The product is available in capsule and powder form. For topical use in pain relief, it is available as a cream, lotion, or gel.

Overdosage
MSM is considered to have very low toxicity. However, doses exceeding 8,000 milligrams per day may cause diarrhea.

NADH (Nicotinamide Adenine Dinucleotide)

Why People Take It

A chemical cousin of vitamin B_3 (niacin), NADH is naturally present in each of the body's cells, where it's needed to trigger conversion of nutrients into the cellular "fuel" adenosine triphosphate (ATP). Proponents of NADH have tested it for several serious diseases, including Parkinson's, Alzheimer's, depression, and chronic fatigue syndrome. However, *controlled* studies (trials comparing patients receiving a drug with others who aren't) have so far been conducted only for chronic fatigue syndrome. The results, while promising, are considered preliminary by experts.

What It Is; How It Works

Because of its role in the synthesis of ATP, NADH is a key factor in the body's production of energy. There is also some evidence that high levels of NADH in the brain may increase production of such chemical messengers as dopamine, norepinephrine, and serotonin. The body produces NADH continuously, using vitamin B_3 as raw material. NADH is also readily available from such dietary sources as fish, poultry, beef, and products made with yeast. Deficiencies of NADH in the United States are almost unknown, except in rare cases of alcoholism.

Research on the use of NADH for treatment of chronic fatigue syndrome has produced encouraging, though not spectacular, results. The study included 26 patients with chronic fatigue, and found that 31 percent of those taking 10 milligrams of NADH daily had fewer symptoms. The researchers theorize that a shortage of ATP may contribute to the symptoms of chronic fatigue, and that the extra NADH works by helping to replenish depleted cellular stores of the compound.

Because Parkinson's disease is caused by a shortage of dopamine at certain locations in the brain, researchers have speculated that NADH's dopamine-boosting effect might relieve the tremors and rigidity the disease produces. Preliminary studies seem to indicate that for many Parkinson's patients this may be true. In one trial of NADH in 885 people with Parkinson's disease, nearly 80 percent showed improvement. (There were, however, no "controls"—patients given no NADH—to provide a basis of comparison for judging the results.)

Since NADH supports production of other chemical messengers in the brain, scientists are also eyeing it for use against Alzheimer's disease and depression. In one small trial, 17 patients suffering from Alzheimer's showed improvement after taking NADH for 8 to 12 weeks. Likewise, a 10-month trial of NADH in 205 depressed patients ended in improvement for 93 percent. But since these studies were small, uncontrolled, and conducted by advocates of NADH, experts say more rigorous testing is needed before any firm conclusions can be drawn.

Avoid if . . .

Given the lack of conclusive research, it would be unwise to use NADH as a replacement for more promising treatments. Although there are no known reasons to avoid the supplement, it's best used as part of an overall treatment plan designed by your doctor.

Special Cautions

Little is known about the effects of long-term, high-dose use of NADH, but excessive use of the related compound nicotinic acid can lead to liver damage, so caution is in order.

Possible Drug Interactions

No drug interactions are known.

Special Information if You Are Pregnant or Breast-feeding

No information is available on the effects of NADH in pregnancy or while breast-feeding. Like any supplement with uncertain effects, it should be avoided during this critical period.

Available Preparations and Dosage

NADH is available in 2.5- and 5-milligram tablets. A typical dosage recommendation is 10 milligrams per day, with water, on an empty stomach. An injectable form is used by physicians to treat complications of alcoholism.

Overdosage

No information is available on overdosage.

Omega-3 Fatty Acids

Why People Take Them

These special fatty acids, found in most cold-water fish, may lower the risk of heart disease. Greenland Inuits have a diet high in fat, but one that is also high in Omega-3s, and they have a far lower incidence of heart disease and far less cholesterol in their blood than the average beef-eating American. In addition, they have lower rates of some cancers and almost no high blood pressure, obesity, arthritis, or diabetes. While there's no proof that Omega-3s are responsible for this situation, proponents consider it more than a coincidence.

Ongoing research suggests that Omega-3 Fatty Acids may also reduce symptoms of bipolar disorder, schizophrenia, and other psychiatric disorders by helping to regulate mood. Some scientists feel there's also a possibility that the Omega-3s can ease the symptoms of arthritis, lupus, and endometriosis, and that they may promote bone growth and fight the brittle-bone disease osteoporosis.

What They Are; How They Work

Omega-3 Fatty Acids are among the highly polyunsaturated fats that tend to keep cholesterol levels in check. Dubbed eicosapentaenoic acid (EPA) and docosahexaenoic acid (DHA), they are found primarily in cold-water fish such as cod, mackerel, sardines, herring, tuna, and salmon. A vegetable product called perilla oil is also richly endowed with these acids, and they can be manufactured by the body, using another fatty acid—alpha linolenic acid (LNA)—as a raw material. Good sources of LNA include flaxseed and canola oils, walnuts, soybeans, spinach, and mustard greens. (For more information on the major sources of Omega-3s, see the separate entries on Fish Oils, Flaxseed Oil, and Perilla Oil.)

EPA and DHA have been shown to lower total cholesterol and triglyceride levels, while raising "good" HDL cholesterol. They also exert a blood-thinning effect by increasing the slipperiness of the blood platelets involved in clot formation. This is thought to discourage the buildup of artery-clogging plaque and reduce the risk of heart attack due to a clot in the coronary arteries. By expanding the blood vessels, EPA may also lower blood pressure in those with hypertension.

Researchers speculate that the Omega-3 Fatty Acids may confer their cardiovascular benefits by displacing another, less beneficial, type of fatty acid called omega-6. Omega-3s also appear to suppress the production of prostaglandins, hormonelike substances that often promote inflammation. It is this property that could make them beneficial to people suffering from inflammatory diseases such as arthritis.

Avoid if . . .

Because of their blood-thinning effects, you should not take Omega-3 supplements if you have a bleeding disorder such as hemophilia or a tendency to hemorrhage.

Special Cautions

If you decide to boost Omega-3 levels by taking fish oil supplements, you should know that cod liver or other fish liver oils are so rich in vitamins A and D that high doses of the oils could cause vitamin toxicity. High doses of fish oil have also been known to increase "bad" LDL cholesterol levels and cause an increase in blood sugar. See the entry on fish oil for more information.

Possible Drug Interactions

If you are taking a blood-thinning drug such as aspirin or Coumadin, check with your doctor before taking Omega-3 supplements, which could further thin the blood.

Special Information if You Are Pregnant or Breast-feeding

During pregnancy, do not take extra Omega-3s in the form of fish oil. High doses (25,000 IU or more) of the vitamin A in fish oil can cause birth defects.

Available Preparations and Dosage

There is no recommended dietary allowance (RDA) for Omega-3 Fatty Acids. To boost your intake, most nutritionists recommend eating fish two or three times a week, rather than taking large amounts of supplements. A 7-ounce serving of salmon or bluefish provides

2.4 grams of Omega-3 acids. The same serving of herring contains 3.2 grams.

To supplement your intake of linolenic acid—and thus the body's supply of Omega-3s—you can also take flaxseed. Typical doses are 35 to 50 grams of crushed seeds or 1 to 2 tablespoonfuls of flaxseed oil daily. To add extra linolenic acid to your diet, make a habit of using canola oil in cooking.

If you use fish oil, flaxseed oil, or perilla oil, remember that these products can quickly become rancid. Store them in air-tight containers kept in the refrigerator.

Overdosage

Excessive intake of Omega-3s can lead to bleeding problems in case of accident or trauma, and may cause anemia in menstruating women. Large doses of fish oil can also lead to problems. See the fish oil entry for additional information.

Ornithine

Why People Take It

By boosting the body's production of human growth hormone, Ornithine is said to yield two major health benefits: a reinvigorated immune system and a leaner, more muscular body.

An amino acid, Ornithine is produced in the body from arginine, a related amino acid with similar properties (see separate entry). Both compounds stimulate synthesis of growth hormone, which in turn is said to promote growth of the white blood cells that patrol the body on search-and-destroy missions against bacteria, viruses, and cancer-causing chemicals. They also aid in healing and repair of damaged tissues. And, in large doses, they are said to promote weight loss by building muscle while burning off extra fat.

Ornithine is one of the raw materials of spermine and spermidine, two compounds that support production of sperm. Some researchers have linked low levels of spermine with poor memory, and suggest that Ornithine supplements could serve as memory boosters. This theory has not yet, however, been verified in clinical trials.

Ornithine also plays a role in the processing of the body's waste products for elimination in the urine, helping to rid the body of toxic ammonia. It supports liver function and helps the liver filter waste products from the blood. Because of its beneficial effect on the liver—it may even help the liver regenerate—Ornithine has been used as a treatment when people with liver disease lapse into coma.

What It Is; How It Works

Ornithine is available in milk products, as well as chicken and other meats. Because the body can produce a certain amount of Ornithine when it's lacking in the diet, it is considered a "nonessential" amino acid. Nevertheless, diets severely deficient in protein may leave the body with a shortage of this important nutrient.

Scientists have yet to conduct the major human trials needed to verify Ornithine's protective effects against germs and toxins. However, tests on laboratory animals have been encouraging. In one animal study, a combination of Ornithine and arginine effectively blocked tumors from forming in mice injected with a cancer-causing virus.

Avoid if . . .

Children should not be given Ornithine supplements due to its impact on growth hormone levels. For the same reason, it should be avoided during pregnancy and breast-feeding. Ornithine and arginine sometimes reactivate latent herpes virus infections; so people who have had brain or ocular herpes must strictly avoid both substances. Ornithine may also aggravate schizophrenia and shouldn't be taken by anyone with this disorder.

Special Cautions

Growth hormone and substances that promote its release, such as Ornithine, can aggravate diabetes; diabetics must use them with care. Although side effects are rare, Ornithine occasionally causes insomnia.

Possible Drug Interactions

No interactions have been reported.

Special Information if You Are Pregnant or Breast-feeding

Because it affects growth hormone, Ornithine should be avoided during pregnancy and breast-feeding.

Available Preparations and Dosage

Ornithine and arginine are typically taken together. Ornithine is available by itself in 500-milligram hard gelatin
capsules. Combination supplements containing 500 milligrams of arginine and 250 milligrams of Ornithine are
also available, reflecting the belief that Ornithine is twice
as potent as arginine. Typical Ornithine doses range from
1,000 to 2,500 milligrams daily; arginine doses are double
those amounts.

Overdosage

Excess growth hormone can make the skin tough and
thick. This problem will disappear when the amount of
growth hormone in the body returns to normal. However, long-term stimulation of growth hormone can lead
to other changes that don't go away, including enlargement of the larynx, deepening of the voice, and over-
grown joints. Excessive growth hormone has also been
linked to certain cases of diabetes (high blood sugar).

Oscillococcinum

Why People Take It

This patented homeopathic remedy is a popular item in
health food stores during flu season. Marketed for the re-

lief of influenza symptoms such as fever, chills, aches, and pains, Oscillococcinum (pronounced o-sill-oh-cox-in-um) is the leading nonprescription remedy for flu symptoms in France, according to Boiron, Inc., the French company that manufactures it. It is also a prime example in the ongoing controversy over homeopathic medicine: its supporters claim it's one of the most scientifically validated of all homeopathic remedies, while debunkers hold it up as a classic example of the reason homeopathy is mere quackery.

What It Is; How It Works

Oscillococcinum is prepared from the heart and liver of wild duck, but like most homeopathic medicines, this one is diluted so many times that a given dose may not contain a single molecule of duck. Following this "law of infinitesimals" is a hallmark of homeopathy, but one that defies the principles of mainstream medical science. Some drugs do work better at lower doses than at higher ones, but none work better when the active ingredient is essentially missing. Why duck liver? Because of another seemingly paradoxical law of homeopathy: "Like cures like" (substances that cause symptoms can cure the same symptoms when taken in small enough doses), and duck organs are claimed to be reservoirs for influenza viruses.

These unscientific-sounding principles have long given skeptics cause to label all homeopathic medicine a fraud, or at best a placebo (a "dummy pill" that works because a patient believes it will). And indeed, past clinical trials of Oscillococcinum, although purporting to prove it effective, have failed to meet rigorous standards of scientific research.

In recent years, however, a few homeopathic products, including Oscillococcinum, have actually performed better than a placebo in a handful of well-conducted clinical trials, the kind in which patients are randomly assigned to the medicine or a placebo without knowing which. In a review of seven such trials of Oscillococcinum, researchers from Memorial Sloan-Kettering Cancer Center found that the product might indeed shorten the duration of flu symptoms (although not by much). The researchers called the evidence promising, but didn't find it strong enough to recommend Oscillococcinum as a first-choice therapy for the flu.

Homeopaths continue to theorize about how their ultra-diluted remedies actually work, suggesting that the water in which the active ingredients are diluted retains some kind of "memory" or energy pattern. Even skeptics agree that if they ever prove their case, the conventional wisdom about how drugs cure disease will be turned on its head.

Avoid if . . .
The makers of Oscillococcinum state that it is safe for people with other medical conditions and free from any side effects—not surprising, its critics would add, for a product that contains virtually no active ingredients.

Special Cautions
Like most homeopathic remedies, Oscillococcinum presents only two risks: wasting money and—if you rely on the product exclusively—losing an opportunity for more effective medical treatment. Since Oscillococcinum is safe and moderately priced by the standards of trendy al-

ternative remedies, there's little to lose by trying it at the first sign of flu and deciding for yourself—provided you don't forgo standard medical care. Be extra cautious if you have other medical conditions that make flu especially dangerous for you. Standard care for the flu starts with immunization shots recommended for high-risk individuals such as the elderly and those with respiratory conditions like asthma. Several prescription medications are also available to tame the symptoms of flu in addition to these old standbys, bed rest and chicken soup.

Possible Drug Interactions

Drug interactions, the manufacturer assures us, are not a problem. Detractors would agree, citing the lack of anything with which a drug could interact.

Special Information if You Are Pregnant or Breast-feeding

The remedy's manufacturer claims that Oscillococcinum may be used by children and pregnant women under a physician's supervision. Given the diluted-to-nothing nature of homeopathic remedies, this is a reasonable assumption.

Available Preparations and Dosage

Like many homeopathic preparations, Oscillococcinum is formulated in tiny pellets for oral dosing. Each dose is packaged in a separate tube; the recommended dosage is one dose every 6 hours for a total of three doses daily, to be taken at the first signs of influenza.

Overdosage

Because this remedy contains no detectable active ingredient, overdosage is not a concern.

PABA (Para-Aminobenzoic Acid)

Why People Take It

Best known as the active ingredient in a variety of sunblock products, PABA has been tried as a remedy for several unusual disorders, but without notable success. It has been studied for the treatment of diseases marked by an abnormal buildup of fibrous tissues, such as scleroderma, but has rarely produced an effect. Some researchers have also reported that it relieves certain skin diseases such as vitiligo, in which the skin loses pigment in patches. Other studies, however, suggest that PABA may actually worsen this disease.

A single study done nearly 60 years ago found PABA useful as a treatment for female infertility, but the results have never been duplicated. It has also been used, but again without much scientific verification, as a treatment for male infertility. Some alternative health authorities claim PABA can darken gray hair in some older adults, though in most trials it has failed to do so. Also unverified are claims that PABA helps to slow aging, support the immune system, treat arthritis and headaches, and relieve constipation.

What It Is; How It Works

PABA is a member of the vitamin B complex. It is required in the formation of folic acid in the body and aids in the breakdown and use of proteins. Through its association with folic acid, it promotes red blood cell formation. It is also said to enhance the effects of cortisone and estrogen by delaying their breakdown in the liver.

A water-soluble vitaminlike substance, PABA is not considered to be an essential human nutrient. However, to the extent that all members of the B complex are needed for maximum effect, PABA may lend support to the other vitamins in the B family.

Under ordinary circumstances, there's no need for extra PABA in the diet. If a shortage does develop, it will be signaled by headaches, fatigue, depression, nervousness, and digestive disturbances. Good sources of PABA include brewer's yeast, bran, wheat germ, eggs, liver, spinach, molasses, and rice.

Avoid if . . .

If you're allergic to sunscreens containing PABA, you should probably avoid PABA supplements.

Special Cautions

High doses of PABA can be fatal, especially in children, and sustained megadosing can cause low blood sugar, rash, fever, and liver damage. Consult with a physician before giving PABA to a child, before taking doses of more than 400 milligrams per day, and before taking PABA preparations for an extended period of time.

Possible Drug Interactions

Do not combine PABA with sulfa drugs, methotrexate, or the antibacterial drug Dapsone; it may interfere with their effects. Because PABA is often one of the ingredients in multivitamin products, be sure to read all your supplement labels.

Special Information if You Are Pregnant or Breast-feeding

PABA spurs production of folic acid, and adequate amounts of folic acid are essential during pregnancy. Nevertheless, the full effects of PABA supplementation during pregnancy are unknown, so it's best to avoid it while pregnant or breast-feeding.

Available Preparations and Dosage

PABA is widely available in strengths ranging from 50 to 1,000 milligrams. It can be purchased by itself, in combination with other B vitamins, and in multivitamin supplements. It's an ingredient in many children's vitamin products.

Typical daily dosages never exceed 400 milligrams, though megadoses of up to 12 grams a day are sometimes prescribed for disorders of the connective tissue and skin. Daily doses above the 400-milligram level should be taken only under a doctor's supervision.

Overdosage

Children have reportedly died from PABA overdoses. Massive doses can damage the liver, heart, and kidneys.

Symptoms include loss of appetite, nausea, vomiting, and shortness of breath.

Pantethine

Why People Take It

Pantethine is a form of pantothenic acid (vitamin B_5) that offers some benefits not available from other forms of the vitamin. In particular, Pantethine has been shown to lower blood cholesterol and triglyceride levels. Some studies have found that it's especially helpful for diabetics, reducing cholesterol without disturbing blood sugar. It appears to be particularly useful for diabetics on dialysis.

Other benefits are less well documented. The substance has been used as a treatment for cataracts and hepatitis A, as a detoxifier of alcohol in the body, and as an immune stimulant, but results have been inconclusive. Most current research focuses on Pantethine's potential value in lowering cholesterol and protecting against cardiovascular disease.

What It Is; How It Works

Pantothenic acid is so common in plants and animals that its name is taken from a Greek word meaning "everywhere." It is necessary for the formation of cell membranes and plays an important role in a variety of the body's metabolic processes. It also aids the healing process and supports the normal functioning of the nervous system. Common in many foods, it is also produced by the bacteria in our intestines. Good dietary sources include blue cheese, brewer's yeast and baker's yeast, eggs, lobster, salmon, all kinds of meats (especially liver), lentils, peanuts, peas, soybeans, sunflower seeds, wheat germ, corn, and whole grain products. Because it's so widely available in common foods, cases of deficiency are rare.

Pantothenic acid (and Pantethine) acts as a coenzyme to facilitate the release of energy from carbohydrates, protein, and fat. It plays an essential role in the body's production of cholesterol and fatty acids. It is also needed in the production of acetylcholine, one of the nervous system's key chemical messengers. It stimulates the adrenal glands to expand the body's supply of cortisone and other steroid hormones, and it promotes red blood cell production. It has an acknowledged role in the healing process, and proponents have suggested that it could be helpful in treating arthritis, premenstrual syndrome, vitiligo (mottled skin), and stress-related conditions. It has also been proposed as a remedy for conditions ranging from gray hair, constipation, aging, and fatigue to allergies, cirrhosis of the liver, and stomach ulcers. However, its therapeutic value for such problems remains to be verified.

Pantethine is metabolized slightly differently than pantothenic acid, and this seems to account for its different effects. Pantethine has been tested for a wide range of conditions, including rheumatoid arthritis, acne, lupus, and sinusitis, but the most promising results have been obtained against high cholesterol and triglycerides. Pantethine supplements have been found to lower "bad" LDL cholesterol and triglyceride levels, and raise "good" HDL cholesterol, perhaps by slowing cholesterol synthesis and speeding up the use of fats for energy. A 1990 study showed an improvement in cholesterol levels in perimenopausal women taking 900 milligrams daily. Another study—of 1,045 diabetics taking an average of 900 milligrams daily—found similar improvements. Importantly, Pantethine is well tolerated by most people, with no significant side effects.

Avoid if . . .
At customary dosage levels, Pantethine is safe for virtually everyone. However, rare allergic reactions have been reported.

Special Cautions
While Pantethine promises substantial benefits without risk of side effects, it would be unwise to view it as a substitute for conventional treatment. If you have a condition such as high cholesterol, Pantethine alone may not solve the problem. Regular medical supervision is essential, whether you use Pantethine or not.

Possible Drug Interactions
Do not take supplemental Pantethine if you are taking levodopa for Parkinson's disease. (It's okay, however, to take Pantethine if you are using a combination of carbidopa and levodopa such as the brand Sinemet.)

Special Information if You Are Pregnant or Breast-feeding

Pantethine requirements tend to rise during pregnancy and breast-feeding. However, it's best to check with your doctor before starting Pantethine or any other supplement during this critical period.

Available Preparations and Dosage

There is no official recommended dietary allowance for pantothenic acid. It's estimated that most adults get 4 to 10 milligrams daily in their diet—an amount sufficient to meet the average daily requirement of 4 to 7 milligrams. Stress, injury, and illness may increase the need for pantothenic acid, and some evidence suggests that use of cigarettes, sulfa drugs, some sleeping pills, estrogen, and alcohol tend to raise the body's requirements.

Proponents of the therapeutic use of Pantethine typically recommend taking 300 milligrams 3 times a day. (Therapeutic doses of pantothenic acid range from 50 to 200 milligrams per day.) Pantethine is available in tablet and capsule form, in a wide variety of strengths. It is also available in combination with pantothenic acid.

Overdosage

Pantethine and pantothenic acid are considered similar in toxicity. Daily doses of 1,000 milligrams or more of pantothenic acid have been taken for months without ill effects. However, megadoses of several grams a day can cause diarrhea and water retention. If you develop such problems, discontinue the supplement.

Pectin

Why People Take It

As a form of dietary fiber, Pectin promises a variety of benefits. Health authorities universally agree that fiber contributes to digestive health. High-fiber, low-calorie foods such as fruits and vegetables, all of which contain at least some Pectin, are recommended for weight loss. Diabetics may benefit from adding it to their diets. In addition, preliminary studies have shown that Pectin, particularly grapefruit pectin, can help to lower cholesterol and reduce the risk of heart disease.

Preparations containing Pectin have proven effective in the treatment of gastroesophageal reflux disease (GERD) and heartburn. It has also been studied as a remedy for ulcers, but was found ineffective. Research has shown that Pectin, as an active ingredient in combination with other medications, is useful in treating diarrhea.

Studies with laboratory animals indicate that modified citrus pectin may help to slow the spread of cancer, particularly prostate and colon cancer. While its effect has not yet been confirmed in humans, Pectin is now being widely recommended to cancer patients, since it's unlikely to cause harm and could prove helpful.

What It Is; How It Works

Pectin is the type of water-soluble fiber that is noted for its ability to reduce cholesterol levels. It helps provide structure to plant cells, and is almost impossible to avoid in any kind of normal diet. Primary sources are citrus fruits, apples, potatoes, peas, beans, and oats. Pectin is widely used by food manufacturers as a gelling agent in jams, jellies, and salad dressings.

Studies have found that Pectin works as a diet aid by helping to slow the emptying of the stomach and inhibiting the absorption of food in the intestines, where it provides bulk but is not itself absorbed. Some health authorities think it may be helpful to diabetics because it slows the rise of blood sugar.

In cancer studies in rats, Pectin appeared to reduce the ability of cancer cells that break off from the main tumor and cling elsewhere in the body—the cancer-spreading process called metastasis. Further studies are under way.

Avoid if . . .

Avoid all fiber supplements if you have an intestinal obstruction or fecal impaction, or have difficulty swallowing. Check with your doctor before taking Pectin if you have a fever or there is blood or mucus in your stools.

Special Cautions

As with any dietary fiber, adding large amounts of Pectin to the diet may cause gas or abdominal distress. Increase your intake of Pectin gradually, and always be sure to get plenty of fluids.

Possible Drug Interactions

Large amounts of Pectin may interfere with the absorption of some drugs. Like other fiber supplements, it should be taken at least 2 hours before or after medications.

Special Information if You Are Pregnant or Breast-feeding

Fiber supplements are not known to be harmful. Still, it's best to check with your doctor before using Pectin while pregnant or breast-feeding.

Available Preparations and Dosage

Pectin, mostly made from citrus fruits or apples, is available in tablet and powder form. Mix the powdered form with water or juice according to the manufacturer's directions and drink it quickly before it gels. To avoid the risk of choking, always take fiber supplements such as Pectin with sufficient liquid, at least an 8-ounce serving.

Pectin is also found as an ingredient in commercial diet preparations, multivitamins, and other food supplements.

Overdosage

An overdose of Pectin won't prove toxic. However, large quantities of fiber taken without sufficient fluids could lead to fecal impaction.

Perilla Oil

Why People Take It

This exotic variety of vegetable oil, native to the Orient, has seized attention in recent years as a rich source of the omega-3 fatty acids said to protect against heart disease. It is now promoted as a stomach-friendly alternative to the sometimes upsetting fish oil supplements that people have traditionally taken to get extra omega-3s.

The omega-3 fatty acids in fish oil have been studied for decades. Many proponents believe that these compounds not only can stave off heart disease but may also discourage some forms of cancer and relieve arthritis. Research on Perilla Oil, on the other hand, is still in its earliest stages, with very few formal trials yet conducted in humans.

Nevertheless, animal experiments have uncovered some tantalizing hints of the oil's potential benefits. There is at least a possibility that it can help relieve allergies and asthma, control excess weight and high blood pressure, reduce blood sugar levels, and fight various inflammatory diseases. None of these effects, however, have been confirmed in large-scale trials.

What It Is; How It Works

Perilla Oil is extracted from the seeds and leaves of the beefsteak plant, an Asian herb that resembles the ornamental coleus found in many Western gardens. The oil, which has a delicate fragrance, has been used for years in Japanese cooking.

The omega-3 fatty acids in Perilla Oil are labeled "essential" because they cannot be made by the body but must come from the diet. Advocates say that they lower the levels of artery-clogging triglycerides (fats) and "bad" LDL cholesterol in the blood, while raising the amount of "good" HDL cholesterol. Omega-3s also appear to discourage heart attacks by preventing unwanted clotting, which can lead to a blockage in the arteries serving the heart.

Some researchers believe that Americans suffer from a relative imbalance between omega-3 fatty acids and their more common counterparts, the omega-6 fatty acids found in products such as corn and safflower oils. High intakes of omega-6 compounds seem to promote clogged arteries and blood clots—the opposite of the effects encountered with omega-3s. While both oils are essential parts of the diet, some researchers suggest reducing omega-6 intake and boosting omega-3 levels until the two are roughly in balance.

Avoid if . . .

Due to one of its ingredients, it's best to avoid Perilla Oil during pregnancy and obtain omega-3s from other sources. (See "Special Information if You Are Pregnant or Breast-Feeding.")

Special Cautions

Because omega-3 fatty acids discourage clotting, excessive levels can lead to bleeding problems in case of an accident or trauma. Overly high intake could also increase the risk of anemia for women who menstruate.

In theory, an excessive increase in omega-3 fatty acids could induce bleeding in the brain, leading to stroke. However, diets high in omega-3 fats have not produced such problems in animal tests.

Certain agents—called ketones—in Perilla Oil have been shown in animal studies to cause allergic reactions, including life-threatening breathing difficulties. In humans, the only reported allergic reactions so far have been in Japan, where 20 to 50 percent of long-term workers in the Perilla industry developed skin irritation on their hands.

Possible Drug Interactions

You should check with your doctor before using Perilla Oil if you are already taking cholesterol-lowering or blood-thinning drugs, including aspirin.

Special Information if You Are Pregnant or Breast-feeding

Lab tests suggest that perillaldehyde, one of the compounds in Perilla Oil, might have damaging effects on a developing baby. Do not use this product during pregnancy. Since we do not know whether it appears in breast milk, it would be wise to avoid it while breast-feeding as well.

Available Preparations and Dosage

There is no recommended dietary allowance for the omega-3 fatty acids. Proponents suggest that a daily intake of 3 to 4 grams of Perilla Oil is sufficient to provide a protective effect against heart disease. Specifically, they recommend 6,000 milligrams of stabilized Perilla Oil capsules a day, which provide 3.3 grams of omega-3 fatty acids.

Because dietary fiber can absorb any fatty acid, some supplement manufacturers recommend taking Perilla Oil at a different time than fiber. To enhance absorption, at least one supplier recommends taking Perilla Oil with a sulfur-containing food such as low-fat cottage cheese. And remember that the body cannot process fatty acids without nutrients such as magnesium, zinc, vitamin B_6, vitamin B_3, and vitamin C.

Protect Perilla Oil from heat and light. To maintain shelf life, refrigerate after opening.

Overdosage
No information on overdosage is available.

Phenylalanine

Why People Take It
Phenylalanine serves as one of the raw materials for three of the nervous system's most important chemical messengers: dopamine, epinephrine, and norepinephrine. The body can also convert it to phenylethylamine,

a mood-boosting substance that's said to have pain-relieving effects as well.

In light of these properties, Phenylalanine has been proposed as a treatment for depression, Parkinson's disease, and chronic-pain conditions such as arthritis. Trials for arthritis have yielded conflicting results, but preliminary trials for depression have proved encouraging. Phenylalanine has also been promoted as an appetite suppressant and sexual stimulant, but its effectiveness for these purposes remains unproven.

What It Is; How It Works

An "essential" amino acid that the body can't manufacture on its own, Phenylalanine is one of the building blocks of protein. There are two types: L-phenylalanine and D-phenylalanine. The L variety occurs naturally in the diet and supports production of dopamine, epinephrine, norepinephrine, and the mood elevator phenylethylamine. The D form of the substance doesn't occur naturally and serves only as a raw material for phenylethylamine. Both forms are created during the commercial manufacturing process and are typically sold in the combined supplement known as DLPA. Products containing the L form only are also available.

Outright deficiencies of L-phenylalanine are rare, but have been known to strike people who don't eat enough protein. (Signs of protein deficiency include a loss of energy and stamina, lowered resistance to infection, slow healing of wounds, weakness, and depression.) Foods rich in L-phenylalanine include almonds and peanuts, bananas and avocados, cheese and cottage cheese, lima beans, nonfat dry milk, pumpkin and sesame seeds, and pickled herring. Phenylalanine is also an ingredient of the popular artificial sweetener aspartame.

Avoid if . . .

Children born without the ability to process Phenylalanine can build up dangerous levels of this amino acid, leading to mental retardation, seizures, extreme hyperactivity, and psychosis. Children with this condition, called phenylketonuria, must follow a special diet designed to supply no more Phenylalanine than necessary, and must be monitored regularly for excess Phenylalanine in the blood.

Special Cautions

If you have high blood pressure, use Phenylalanine cautiously; it may aggravate this condition. High doses can also cause anxiety; if you're subject to anxiety attacks, it's wise to keep your doses low.

The combination supplement DLPA occasionally causes mild nausea, heartburn, or headache. Because it can have significant effects on mood, it's best to use this type of Phenylalanine only under a doctor's supervision.

Possible Drug Interactions

Do not combine Phenylalanine supplements with drugs known as MAO inhibitors, including the antidepressants Nardil and Parnate.

Special Information if You Are Pregnant or Breast-feeding

Phenylalanine supplements are not recommended during pregnancy and breast-feeding.

Available Preparations and Dosage

The combination supplement DLPA is available in tablet and capsule form. It has been used in doses ranging from 75 to 1,500 milligrams per day. Discuss dosage with your doctor.

The estimated adult daily requirement for L-phenylalanine and the related amino acid tyrosine combined is approximately 7 milligrams per pound of body weight. Infants require almost 9 times that amount; children need 10 milligrams per pound. Most people fulfill these requirements through diet alone, but commercial L-phenylalanine supplements are available in capsule and tablet form. Follow the manufacturer's dosage instructions, and do not take the supplement with other amino acids or protein foods. L-phenylalanine is most effective if taken on an empty stomach prior to meals. Vitamin B_6 is said to enhance its absorption.

Overdosage

Doses of 1,500 milligrams or less are generally considered safe. However, very high doses can affect your blood pressure and even cause migraines. Check with your doctor if you suspect an overdose.

Phosphatidylcholine

Why People Take It

Two potential benefits have attracted interest in Phosphatidylcholine: its impact on cholesterol levels and its effect on memory loss. Of the two, only its ability to reduce serum cholesterol has received a tentative thumbs-up from researchers.

Several studies have found, for instance, that lecithin, a food supplement rich in Phosphatidylcholine, may lower serum cholesterol by 18 percent. Similarly, Russian investigators have found that a supplement containing Phosphatidylcholine and several related compounds produced significant reductions in total serum cholesterol, triglycerides, and LDL cholesterol—the "bad" variety most closely linked to clogged arteries and heart disease. The improvements were equivalent to those seen in patients taking high doses of nicotinic acid, a form of the B vitamin niacin that's been proven effective in combating heart disease. And unlike high doses of niacin, Phosphatidylcholine had no negative effect on the liver.

More important than Phosphatidylcholine's ability to lower cholesterol is the fact that it may provide direct relief of angina (chest pain due to clogged coronary arteries), reducing both the number and the intensity of attacks. Scientists studying lecithin have found that it may also reduce clumping of platelets in the blood, another phenomenon that probably contributes to heart disease and circulatory diseases of the arms and legs. Platelets normally clump together to stop the bleeding from a cut, but if they form clots within the bloodstream, they can promote a dangerous blockage. In one experiment, investigators gave 12 grams of lecithin a day for three months to patients at risk of heart attacks and found that, in addition to lowering cholesterol, the supplement decreased platelet stickiness.

Hopes that Phosphatidylcholine might combat memory loss have been based on its ability to increase levels of acetylcholine in the brain. This important chemical messenger appears to play a role in maintaining memory, and has been found to be in short supply in Alzheimer's patients. Unfortunately, an analysis of 11 carefully controlled clinical experiments with lecithin supplements was unable to detect any significant benefit. The supplement may have very modest effects on patients with impaired thinking or dementia, but it doesn't seem to yield any major improvement.

Similarly, some experts once believed that Phosphatidylcholine might relieve the symptoms of tardive dyskinesia, a severe neurological disorder that's brought on by long-term use of certain antipsychotic drugs. But when schizophrenic patients suffering from the signs and symptoms of the disorder—involuntary movements of the muscles of the face, mouth, and cheeks—were put on lecithin or related compounds, they experienced only slight improvement.

What It Is; How It Works

Phosphatidylcholine is a combination of choline, fatty acids, glycerol, and phosphorus. It is one of several phosphorus-based compounds contained in lecithin, a naturally occurring substance derived from beef liver, eggs, soybeans, and peanuts. Lecithin products are generally composed of from 5 to 30 percent Phosphatidylcholine.

Choline, the most important ingredient in Phosphatidylcholine, constitutes about 13 percent of the total. It has recently been classified as an essential nutrient by the National Academy of Sciences. (See entry on choline.)

Avoid if . . .

Phosphatidylcholine is generally considered safe.

Special Cautions

High doses of choline can cause overstimulation, muscle tension, and digestive upsets. You'd need to take extremely large doses of Phosphatidylcholine to achieve a similar effect, but cases have been reported.

Possible Drug Interactions

It's best to avoid choline-containing supplements if you're taking a prescription drug such as scopolamine (an antinausea medication) that works by blocking the effects of acetylcholine.

Special Information if You Are Pregnant or Breast-feeding

For healthy women, choline supplements are not recommended during pregnancy and breast-feeding.

Available Preparations and Dosage

Phosphatidylcholine supplements typically come in capsule and powder form. Potency ranges from 20 to 100 percent.

Dosage recommendations for formulations containing 55 percent Phosphatidylcholine range from 1,000 to 2,000 milligrams daily, supplying from 72 to 144 milligrams of choline. The National Academy of Sciences estimates that adults need 425 to 550 milligrams of choline a day to stay healthy. A typical diet usually supplies the full basic requirement.

Overdosage

The upper tolerable limit of choline is 3.5 grams a day. (It takes approximately 27 grams of Phosphatidylcholine to supply this amount.) Dosages above this level may bring on dizziness, nausea, diarrhea, cramps, and a fishy body odor.

Phytoestrogens

Why People Take Them

Phytoestrogens, the hormonelike compounds found in a variety of beans, fruits, and herbs, appear to offer many of the same benefits as human estrogen, the hormone that governs the menstrual cycle. Researchers have found, for instance, that women who eat Phytoestrogen-rich soybean products have longer cycles, strongly suggesting that the foods mimic the action of the human hormone.

Similarly, a recent study of women at menopause, when estrogen levels decline, found that adding daily servings of isolated soy protein to their diets reduced the number of hot flashes they experienced. And since neither the volunteers participating in this trial nor the researchers themselves knew who was getting the soy and who was getting an inactive substitute—an experiment referred to as a double-blind study—it's unlikely that the results were influenced by prior belief in the benefits of soy.

Phytoestrogens from other sources offer similar benefits. Studies conducted with the phytoestrogen-laden herb black cohosh found that taking either two tablets or 40 drops of a black cohosh extract twice daily relieved the symptoms of menopause.

Nor are the benefits limited to postmenopausal relief. Other researchers have discovered that women who eat large amounts of Phytoestrogen-rich foods are less likely to develop breast cancer. And scientists have noted that men—who also respond to estrogen—suffer less prostate cancer if they follow a vegetarian diet or live in preindustrial African or Asian communities, where people rely more heavily on Phytoestrogen-rich fruits and vegetables. (Researchers have not, however, ruled out the possibility that some other difference in diet or lifestyle may account for the lower rate.)

After menopause, estrogen replacement therapy staves

off osteoporosis and heart disease, and some studies suggest a similar role for Phytoestrogens. In keeping with this line of reasoning, the U.S. Food and Drug Administration, on the basis of convincing evidence, has recently given food manufacturers permission to state on their labels that soy foods can reduce the threat of heart disease.

What They Are; How They Work

Phytoestrogens are actually a family of compounds, including isoflavones and lignins. Isoflavones are found primarily in legumes like soybeans, peas, and beans, while lignins are found in nuts, cereals, berries, and various other fruits and vegetables. Investigators have found more than twenty types of Phytoestrogens in vegetation. In some plants, scientists have isolated hormones identical to those found in the animal kingdom. These plants include pomegranates, green beans, dates, hops, licorice, and apples.

The effect of Phytoestrogens depends in part on how much estrogen the body is already producing and how saturated its estrogen receptor sites have become. If estrogen levels are low, as in menopause, empty estrogen receptor sites can be filled with Phytoestrogens, which then exert a weak estrogenlike effect. If estrogen levels are high, as in premenstrual syndrome (PMS) and endometriosis, then Phytoestrogens that bind with the receptors will displace regular estrogen, moderating its effects. Phytoestrogens may also trick the hypothalamus and pituitary glands, which regulate female hormones, into thinking the body has enough estrogen, thus reducing internal estrogen production and the health risks—such as uterine cancer and possibly breast cancer—posed by high levels of the more potent human hormone.

Avoid if . . .
Phytoestrogens are generally considered safe for everyone.

Special Cautions
Although Phytoestrogen-rich foods present no problems, certain extracts demand caution. For instance, Germany's Commission E, a government group that studies and regulates herbal medicines, recommends that use of black cohosh be limited to six months.

Possible Drug Interactions
Dong quai, a Chinese herb that contains Phytoestrogens, also contains coumarin, which acts as a blood thinner. Persons on anticoagulant drugs may therefore want to avoid combining the herb with their medication for fear that it will have an additive effect, increasing the risk of bleeding.

Black cohosh should be used cautiously by patients taking medications to lower their blood pressure because the herb itself has been reported to lower blood pressure, and the combined effect could cause one's pressure to drop too low. The resulting hypotension can cause dizziness and fainting.

Special Information if You Are Pregnant or Breast-feeding
While there are no specific precautions for Phytoestrogens as a group, experts warn that black cohosh, a rich source of these compounds, should be avoided in pregnancy. That's the case because the herb has the potential

to act like oxytocin, a hormone made by the pituitary gland that increases uterine contractions.

Available Preparations and Dosage

Herbal extracts such as black cohosh and dong quai are available in tablet, capsule, and liquid form. Follow the manufacturer's directions for proper dosage.

With soy isoflavones, some studies suggest that 40 to 80 milligrams daily may relieve hot flashes, or even improve cholesterol levels. Soy products such as tofu (soybean curd), tempeh (soybean cake), and roasted soy nuts contain about 40 milligrams per half cup. A full cup of soy milk provides the same amount. Two servings a day may be needed to relieve menopausal symptoms.

Overdosage

No information is available.

Phytosterols

Why People Take Them

These plant-based analogs of cholesterol have assumed a significant role in the ongoing battle against heart disease. Two of the most thoroughly studied Phytosterols, sitosterol and sitostanol, have been shown to lower artery-clogging serum cholesterol levels and are now included in a variety of "designer foods." Several "heart-healthy" margarines and salad dressings rely on these Phytosterols to achieve their effect.

Clinical studies have found that 2 to 4 grams a day of sitosterol or sitostanol can lower blood levels of "bad" LDL cholesterol by as much as 14 percent. In one study, for example, a third of a group of women who had previously suffered heart attacks were able to drive their LDL levels down to less than 100 milligrams per deciliter, which is considered safe. Similarly, in another investigation one of the "heart-healthy" margarines lowered total serum cholesterol by about 24 points. To put these numbers into perspective, experts estimate that every 1 percent drop in serum cholesterol yields a 2 percent decline in your risk of coronary heart disease.

Even if you're already eating a low-fat, low-cholesterol diet, chances are that adding Phytosterol-containing products to your menu will still be beneficial. Researchers have found that volunteers who eat a low-fat diet plus Phytosterols have lower serum LDL levels than those who combine the same products with a higher-fat diet.

Researchers have also shown that Phytosterols offer added benefits when combined with cholesterol-lowering prescription drugs. When patients were given Pravachol alone, for example, their LDL levels dropped by 38 percent, while adding Phytosterols to their regimen caused their lipid levels to plummet 44 percent.

Still, it's worth keeping one caveat in mind: While there's little doubt that Phytosterols reduce cholesterol levels, researchers have yet to formally prove that products containing these substances lower the odds of a heart attack or reduce the death rate from heart disease.

In unrelated research, scientists have also found that Phytosterols often relieve the symptoms of prostate enlargement (benign prostatic hyperplasia). In four separate clinical studies involving over 500 men with enlarged prostate, sitosterol, given at a dose of 60 to 195 milligrams per day, significantly reduced urinary symptoms. The men were less likely to have to get up in the middle of the night to urinate and were able to more fully empty their bladders.

What They Are; How They Work

Because these plant-derived compounds have a chemical structure similar to cholesterol, they partially block the absorption of cholesterol in the gastrointestinal tract. They also interfere with the reabsorption of cholesterol that has been secreted into the digestive tract in bile. The drop in cholesterol uptake indirectly brings about a reduction in blood levels of LDL cholesterol.

Avoid if . . .

There's no known reason to avoid Phytosterols.

Special Cautions

Aside from some mild constipation, there have been no reported side effects from Phytosterol-enriched foods. Some experts suspect, however, that they may interfere with the absorption of fat-soluble nutrients like beta-carotene. As a result, some products are fortified with beta-carotene to avert any possible deficiency.

Possible Drug Interactions
No interactions have been reported.

Special Information if You Are Pregnant or Breast-feeding
Adequate cholesterol is essential for the developing baby. While Phytosterols are not known to cause any direct harm, attempts to achieve very low cholesterol levels are unwise during pregnancy.

Available Preparations and Dosage
To lower cholesterol levels, the usual recommendation is 1 to 2 tablespoons daily of a Phytosterol-enriched margarine such as Benecol or Take Control.

Overdosage
Oral doses as high as 3 grams have not caused serious side effects.

Potassium Glycerophosphate

Why People Take It
Promoted as the most readily absorbed and easily metabolized form of potassium available, Potassium Glycerophosphate has been adopted by fitness enthusiasts as an aid to

better, harder training. Overexertion and excessive sweating can deplete the body's potassium stores, which in turn results in weakness, fatigue, and muscle cramps. Proponents say that potassium supplements help to prevent these unpleasant aftereffects of intensive training.

There are also claims that the glycerophosphate in this product helps the body produce adenosine triphosphate (ATP), the chemical that fuels the muscles. Glycerophosphate is also believed to aid exercisers by eliminating lactic acid, a by-product of muscular activity that can cause tired, achy muscles and muscle spasms. However, there have been no clinical trials to verify these theories.

There is, of course, no question that Potassium Glycerophosphate can remedy potassium deficiency. Potassium is needed for the proper functioning of the heart, muscles, kidneys, and nerves, and excessively low levels can cause widespread muscular malfunctions, impair the kidneys, and trigger irregular heartbeats. In addition, a shortage of potassium, combined with an oversupply of sodium, can lead to high blood pressure. Studies have shown that potassium intake can reduce the need for blood pressure medicine in people with low potassium levels. Moreover, some animal and human studies have shown that potassium supplements can reduce the risk of stroke.

What It Is; How It Works

Potassium Glycerophosphate is an organically bound compound of potassium and glycerophosphate. Both ingredients are part of any ordinary diet. Potassium, a mineral and an electrolyte, is found in fruits, vegetables, nuts, whole grains, and dairy products. Glycerophosphate can be obtained from poultry, meat, fish, cereal, and dairy products.

Potassium Glycerophosphate is classified therapeutically as a tonic. It easily passes through cell walls, and thus is able to aid in the conduction of nerve impulses that regulate the heartbeat and cause muscle contractions.

Avoid if . . .

There is no reason to avoid Potassium Glycerophosphate. The dietary supplement is "generally recognized as safe" by the U.S. Food and Drug Administration.

Special Cautions

Strictly limit the size of your doses. Excessive levels of potassium (hyperkalemia) can disrupt the heartbeat, cause paralysis in the arms and legs, and produce a serious drop in blood pressure. The risk of hyperkalemia is small, since excess potassium is usually eliminated quickly in the urine. However, a buildup is possible in someone suffering kidney problems, gastrointestinal bleeding, rapid protein breakdown, or a major infection.

Possible Drug Interactions

Do not combine Potassium Glycerophosphate with drugs that control spasms, such as Bentyl, Donnatal, and Lomotil. Be cautious if you are taking a high blood pressure medicine categorized as an ACE inhibitor (for example, Capoten or Vasotec) or a potassium-sparing diuretic (Aldactone or Midamor). These drugs can drive up your potassium level. If you're unsure about any of the drugs you're taking, check with your doctor before taking any extra potassium.

Special Information if You Are Pregnant or Breast-feeding
At ordinary intake levels, Potassium is generally considered safe during pregnancy and nursing.

Available Preparations and Dosage
There is no official recommended dietary allowance for potassium. Your needs vary according to the amount of salt you use. However, for general purposes, many experts peg the minimum daily requirement at roughly 2,000 to 2,500 milligrams. Since a normal diet can supply as much as 6,000 milligrams a day, supplements are usually unnecessary. They are typically recommended only when certain medical conditions or prescription drugs deplete the body's supply.

Potassium Glycerophosphate is most often found as an ingredient within a combination supplement product. Supplements that contain Potassium Glycerophosphate are available in capsule, tablet, powder, and liquid form.

Overdosage
A severe overdose can lead to convulsions, coma, and even cardiac arrest. Seek emergency treatment immediately if you notice such early warning signs of overdose as muscle weakness or paralysis, fast or irregular heartbeat, or blood in your stool.

Pregnenolone

Why People Take It

Promoted as the "mother of all hormones" because it serves as a raw material for many other steroid hormones, Pregnenolone isn't known to have any specific functions of its own. Nevertheless, advocates of Pregnenolone and its offspring, DHEA, refer to them as "superhormones," suggesting that they can be used as over-the-counter solutions to conditions such as depression, rheumatoid arthritis, Alzheimer's disease, multiple sclerosis, immune disorders, premenstrual syndrome (PMS), and the symptoms of menopause.

To date, none of these claims has been verified in reliable clinical trials. However, Pregnenolone is classified as a neurosteroid—a chemical known to modify mood and behavior—and some researchers believe that it does have a beneficial modifying effect on the activity of chemical messengers (neurotransmitters) and receptors in the brain, helping to balance and stabilize brain function.

In one small study of young men, it seems to have improved sleep and decreased the frequency of night waking. A World War II–era study of fatigued army pilots suggested that it may also play a role in helping the body deal with the effects of stress. Other research, conducted nearly 50 years ago, indicated that injectable Pregnenolone might be helpful in the treatment of arthritic and rheumatologic conditions such as lupus, psoriasis, and scleroderma.

More recently, studies of Pregnenolone done on laboratory animals have demonstrated its ability to enhance memory. One study that tested Pregnenolone along with an anti-inflammatory and an immune system enhancer found that the combination helped improve motor function in rats with spinal cord injury. However, neither of these properties has yet been verified in humans.

Indeed, scientists still aren't certain whether taking supplementary Pregnenolone has *any* significant beneficial effect. What we do know is that Pregnenolone is a powerful substance that could affect the entire hormone balance of the body. Further research is being conducted, but until more is known, the safest course is to take Pregnenolone only with great caution and under a doctor's supervision.

What It Is; How It Works

Pregnenolone is a natural substance manufactured in the body from cholesterol and found in high concentrations in the brain and other nerve tissues. Pregnenolone sits at the beginning of the steroid assembly line, with a number of other hormones proceeding from it, including dehydroepiandrosterone (DHEA), progesterone, estrogen, and testosterone. While it seems to serve primarily as a source material for these hormones, some health authorities believe that it also has a balancing effect, regulating levels as needed.

Various studies measuring Pregnenolone levels found decreased amounts in people with low thyroid function and increased amounts in those with an overactive thyroid. People with depression also have unusually low levels. Reduced levels have also been linked to conditioned fear response and social isolation in animal studies.

Pregnenolone levels also decline with age, and promoters suggest that certain disease processes—and even aging itself—are "caused" by a shortage of this hormone. However, a variety of body chemicals diminish as we grow older and so far scientists have been unable to single out any specific culprits. On the other hand, they *do* know that trying to restore hormonal levels to those of our youth may have unintended consequences. Estrogen replacement therapy, for example, was prescribed as a menopausal treatment for decades before scientists discovered that it could dramatically increase a woman's risk of certain cancers.

Some researchers also warn that taking Pregnenolone as a dietary supplement could have an inhibitory effect on the body's ability to manufacture its own supply. It's not known whether this is true, but there's no question that the body is in a constant balancing act to keep hormones at an optimal level. Adding Pregnenolone may upset this balance in ways we don't yet understand.

Avoid if . . .

Because of its potential impact on the nervous system, do not take Pregnenolone if you have a history of seizures. Also avoid it if you are at high risk of hormone-dependent cancers such as cancer of the breast, uterus, ovaries, or prostate.

Special Cautions

If you have any kind of glandular disorder, be sure to check with your doctor before taking Pregnenolone. And remember that the long-term effects of this hormonal supplement remain unknown.

Possible Drug Interactions

Do not combine Pregnenolone with the antiseizure drug Neurontin or other drugs chemically similar to the neurotransmitter GABA. Remember that Pregnenolone may also affect the action of hormonal medications such as progesterone, testosterone, estrogen, and oral contraceptives, and may require a reduction in the dose of any DHEA supplement you may be taking.

Special Instructions if You Are Pregnant or Breast-feeding

Because of its hormonal effects, do not take Pregnenolone while pregnant or breast-feeding.

Available Preparations and Dosage

Pregnenolone is available from natural supplement suppliers in capsules of 10 to 150 milligrams. There is little agreement over the proper dosage. While some manufacturers promote taking as much as 500 milligrams per day, others advise taking no more than 5 milligrams— and many experts recommend avoiding it entirely. At the very least, if you want to experiment with this product, seek the advice of a physician who is familiar with natural supplements.

Overdosage
No information on overdosage is available.

Proline

Why People Take It

This amino acid supplement is sold primarily as a tonic for muscles, tendons, and joints, and as a remedy for soft-tissue injuries. It's an ingredient in a variety of combination supplements that claim to help build muscle tissue, preserve lean body mass (muscle) during bodybuilding and weight-loss programs, reinforce connective tissue, improve skin health, give an energy boost, promote a healthy heart, decrease blood pressure, and improve memory and mental sharpness.

To the extent that all amino acids are needed for the production of human protein, Proline does in fact build muscle—but probably no more so than would a well-balanced meal. Clinical trials of amino acids in the same category as Proline have failed to uncover any effect on muscle after exercise. There are also no scientific studies confirming the other benefits claimed for this product.

What It Is; How It Works

Proline is one of the "nonessential" amino acids that the body can manufacture on its own if it's lacking in the diet. Proline is also available in dairy products, eggs, meat, poultry, seafood, and nuts.

Athletes and bodybuilders are interested in amino acids such as Proline because these nutrients are needed to build and maintain virtually all the body's tissues, including the muscles. A deficiency of amino acids (or the protein in which they're contained) can stunt growth in children and sap vigor, stamina, and resistance in adults. Hair, nails, skin, and muscles are all adversely affected.

However, extra amino acids won't necessarily give muscles a boost. (Sufficient calorie intake combined with regular exercise is what ultimately builds muscle.) Excess protein is either converted to energy or stored as fat—and because waste products from this conversion are eliminated in the urine, too much protein intake can put a strain on the kidneys and liver. Excess protein consumption also slows the absorption of needed calcium.

Proline has also sparked interest as a potential remedy for joint problems. It's a major component of collagen, the fibrous protein that makes up bone, joint-cushioning cartilage, tendons, and other connective tissue. Although advocates of Proline supplementation are convinced that it can encourage collagen maintenance and repair, there's no solid evidence supporting this view. At this point, scientists don't fully understand what governs collagen synthesis or its breakdown in the human body.

Avoid if . . .

It's best to avoid Proline supplements if you have kidney or liver problems, or a rare condition called prolinemia, type II. This disorder defeats the body's ability to process Proline, and can lead to convulsions and mental retardation.

Special Cautions

The U.S. Food and Drug Administration recognizes Proline as a generally safe dietary supplement when used in accordance with good manufacturing and dietary practices. However, there have been reports of serious reactions to commercial amino acid supplements. Since these products contain as many as fifteen amino acids, it's not known which ingredient, or combination of ingredients, might be at fault.

Remember, too, that amino acid supplements and excessively high intakes of protein can increase calcium loss and put an added burden on the kidneys. Also, the effects of amino acid supplements on the endocrine system—the pituitary, thyroid, and adrenal glands—have not been fully investigated and can't be conclusively judged safe.

Possible Drug Interactions

Tetracycline may reduce absorption of amino acids.

Special Information if You Are Pregnant or Breast-feeding

There is no information on the effect of Proline supplements during pregnancy. Especially at this critical juncture, it's best to avoid any medication that isn't absolutely necessary for your health.

Available Preparations and Dosage

Proline supplements are available in capsule, tablet, and powder form. There are no official recommended dietary allowances for nonessential amino acids such as Proline. Follow the manufacturer's recommendations and avoid sustained megadosing.

Overdosage

Although no specific information is available, even high doses are unlikely to cause any severe problems.

PS (Phosphatidylserine)

Why People Take It

Phosphatidylserine is used to combat memory loss and improve cognitive performance in people with age-related decreases in mental function. It is taken primarily by elderly people with depression, senile dementia, and Alzheimer's disease.

In addition to improved mental performance in people on PS, research has documented positive changes in behavior, such as better social interactions and cooperation with caregivers. Studies have also found beneficial changes in anxiety levels and depression among elderly women taking PS. And there is some evidence that PS can help the body deal with some of the damaging biochemical effects of stress.

Most of what is known about PS comes from studies using a form made from cow brain. Since the scare over "mad cow disease" (bovine spongiform encephalopathy), manufacturers have stopped using cow brain and are now experimenting with supplements made from soy. Medical authorities believe that soy-based PS confers the same benefits as the version derived from cows, but this has yet to be conclusively confirmed.

What It Is; How It Works

PS is a naturally occurring phospholipid produced in the body and found in every cell. Composed primarily of essential fatty acids, phospholipids play a major role in building cell membranes and maintaining their flexibility. PS is particularly abundant in nerve cell membranes, including the junctures where one cell passes a message along to the next (the synapses). The performance of the synapses is believed to decline with age, and researchers believe that PS works by improving their fluidity and integrity. Some animal studies suggest that PS not only maintains healthy brain function but may also help restore damaged brain networks. The beneficial effects of PS on stress are thought to result from its ability to reduce levels of the hormone cortisol, which is produced during periods of extreme stress.

Some people, especially those with age-related mental decline, may have difficulty synthesizing adequate amounts of PS. A deficiency in the building blocks that make up PS could also lead to a shortage. The raw materials needed to assure an ample supply include essential fatty acids, folic acid, and vitamin B_{12}. PS itself is available from only one dietary source—lecithin—and even there is found in only small amounts.

One drawback of PS supplementation is its cost. The daily doses recommended for treatment of age-associated mental decline can cost as much as $100 per month. If this is more than you want to spend, nutritional authorities suggest that maintaining an adequate supply of the raw materials needed to synthesize PS provides a cheaper alternative.

Avoid if . . .
There is no known reason to avoid this natural phospholipid.

Special Cautions
PS per se is generally regarded as safe. However, due to concerns over "mad cow disease," be sure to check the label and make certain that the product is soy-derived.

Possible Drug Interactions
There are no known interactions with PS.

Special Information if You Are Pregnant or Breast-feeding
PS supplements have not been tested for safety during pregnancy. Since the supplements are used primarily for age-related dementia, there's no good reason to risk taking them while pregnant or breast-feeding.

Available Preparations and Dosage
If nutritional deficiencies result in a shortage of PS, your doctor may recommend PS supplementation. The product

is available in 100-milligram capsules. Manufacturers typically recommend a dosage of 300 milligrams per day, taken with meals.

Overdosage
No information on overdosage is available.

Pycnogenol

Why People Take It
Pycnogenol, an extract of pine bark and/or grape seed, is rich in proanthocyanidins, a group of potent antioxidants that reduce the buildup of toxic wastes in the body. The proanthocyanidins, also found in grape seed extract (see separate entry), are used to treat vein and capillary disorders, including varicose veins, retinal degeneration, swelling, and a tendency to bruise easily.

Thanks to its antioxidant properties, Pycnogenol may also reduce the risk of heart disease, and some proponents suggest it may even protect against cancer. It has also been said to relieve conditions such as tendinitis and arthritis by strengthening collagen and elastin, two building blocks of the body's connective tissue.

Although there is a small body of valid scientific research to support some of these claims—particularly the product's effect on heart disease—you should know that Pycnogenol has also been a magnet for quack "cure-all" claims and multilevel distributorship schemes. Most recently, the Federal Trade Commission ordered one Pycnogenol distributor to cease its unsupported claims that the product can cure attention deficit hyperactivity disorder in children.

What It Is; How it Works

Although derived from humble stuff like grape seeds and pine bark, proanthocyanidins carry an impressive biochemical résumé. These pigments, also found in cranberries and tea, belong to a family of plant-based compounds, or phytochemicals, called flavonoids. The antioxidant activity of proanthocyanidins is especially powerful when these compounds are bound together in a form called oligomeric proanthocyanidin complexes, or OPCs. The French biochemist who developed a patented process for extracting OPCs from pine bark and grape seeds coined the name Pycnogenol for the resulting substance. The name's trademark status is still under dispute, but is used generically by many leading supplement manufacturers. Grape seed extract supplements, which supply OPCs that seem to work as well as those in pine bark extract, tend to carry a lower price tag.

Antioxidants are chemicals that bind with and eliminate products of oxidation called free radicals. Unstable free-radical molecules can combine with a variety of compounds within the body, causing damage that can lead to anything from cancer to coronary heart disease.

Reputable research on Pycnogenol has verified a variety of effects that may stem from its antioxidant or other, less well-understood properties. It acts as a vasodilator, opening blood vessels wider, and it reduces the oxidation of "bad" LDL cholesterol—a key step in the buildup that clogs arteries and leads to heart disease. It also may protect against excessive blood clotting. In a study of smokers, a single high dose of Pycnogenol (200 milligrams) worked better than aspirin in reversing the tendency of platelets to clump together (a clot-forming risk), without the bleeding risk associated with aspirin use.

Some studies suggest that Pycnogenol may also increase the action of vitamin C and E in the body by protecting them from oxidative breakdown. In laboratory studies of mice, Pycnogenol has enhanced immune system activity.

Avoid if . . .
Pycnogenol has been used since the 1950s and appears to be relatively safe for everyone.

Special Cautions
At ordinary dosage levels, Pycnogenol seems to cause no problems.

Possible Drug Interactions
No interactions have been reported. However, if you are taking any other medication for heart disease or vascular conditions, it's a good idea to alert your doctor before taking Pycnogenol or other OPC supplements.

Special Information if You Are Pregnant or Breast-feeding
There is little reliable information on the effect of Pycnogenol and OPCs on a developing baby. Since a temporary interruption of therapy won't permanently damage

your health, your wisest course is to avoid these products during pregnancy and breast-feeding.

Available Preparations and Dosage

It is available in capsules ranging from 30 to 100 milligrams. Doses used in trials showing benefits to the venous system have ranged from as little as two 50-milligram tablets a day to as much as 300 milligrams a day. Optimal dosage levels remain unknown.

Overdosage

OPCs are water-soluble nutrients, so excessive amounts are eliminated in urine. There are no well-recognized symptoms or dangers associated with Pycnogenol overdosage.

Pyroglutamate

Why People Take It

Like dietary supplements such as choline and DMAE (dimethylaminoethanol), Pyroglutamate is prized as a potential memory-booster. Also known as pyroglutamic acid and pyrrolidone carboxylic acid (PCA), it is said to increase alertness, concentration, and recall.

There is at least some justification for these claims.

Animal studies have demonstrated Pyroglutamate's ability to raise levels of acetylcholine, one of the key chemical messengers in the brain. And in human trials, it has reportedly reduced memory deficits caused by alcohol, the normal aging process, and multi-infarct dementia.

On the other hand, because of Pyroglutamate's effect on memory, some advocates have also promoted it as an antiaging remedy, with the ability to boost intelligence and postpone or even reverse the normal aging of the brain. This sort of proposition is pure speculation at present, still in need of scientific testing and verification.

What It Is; How It Works

Pyroglutamate is an amino acid found in large concentrations in the brain and cerebrospinal fluid, where it contributes to the chain of chemical reactions that ends in the production of acetylcholine. It is supplied naturally in the diet by vegetables, fruits, dairy products, and meat.

The exact mechanism by which Pyroglutamate may enhance cognitive function is not known. However, its ability to boost output of acetylcholine is thought to be at least part of the answer. The picture is unclear because acetylcholine plays a variety of roles throughout the body, and because older adults often suffer from a shortage of several neurotransmitters in the brain.

Avoid if . . .

Because of the potentially stimulative effects of supplements that boost acetylcholine levels, it might be wise to avoid Pyroglutamate if you suffer from convulsions or bipolar disorder.

Special Cautions

In 1998, the U.S. Food and Drug Administration issued a warning about over-the-counter products that list as one of their ingredients pyroglutamic acid or arginine pyroglutamate (a compound combining Pyroglutamate and the nonessential amino acid arginine). The agency had received reports of nausea, vomiting, headache, rectal rash, and bloody stools in association with such products. However, it's not known whether the Pyroglutamate in the products was the component at fault.

Possible Drug Interactions

There are no reports of interactions with other supplements or drugs.

Special Information if You Are Pregnant or Breast-feeding

Although Pyroglutamate is a normal part of our diet and presumably poses no threat during pregnancy, it's always a good idea to consult with your doctor before using any supplement.

Available Preparations and Dosage

Pyroglutamate is available in tablet, capsule, and powder form. A typical dosage recommendation is 500 milligrams once or twice a day. The dosage for arginine pyroglutamate preparations is similar.

Advocates often recommend combining Pyroglutamate with choline and other supplements meant to enhance production of acetylcholine.

Overdosage

No information on overdosage is available.

Pyruvate

Why People Take It

Pyruvate is promoted as a weight loss aid. In some studies, people taking very high doses of the substance along with a low-fat diet and exercise have experienced a slight reduction in weight and body fat. However, diet and exercise alone are capable of trimming away excess pounds, and Pyruvate suppliers generally recommend much lower doses, so proof of the product's effectiveness is somewhat less than conclusive.

One study also found that, when people stop dieting, they tend to regain a little less weight if they continue taking this supplement. Advocates make a variety of other claims as well. They say that Pyruvate decreases appetite, increases the metabolism, improves heart function, reduces cholesterol, and combats free radicals. Some recommend it as an endurance booster during exercise. However, none of these claims has been verified.

What It Is; How It Works

Pyruvate is a substance created by the body as one of the steps in the production of energy. Pyruvate is also found in some foods, including red apples, dark beer, red wine, and some types of cheese.

The cells in the body release energy by breaking apart the chemical bonds in carbohydrates, proteins, and fats. During this process, a series of chemicals are formed and transformed. Pyruvate, also called pyruvic acid, is created early in the process. Later, it's broken down further in the process of producing ATP (adenosine triphosphate), the energy molecule that fuels all of the body's activities.

It is unclear how (or even if) Pyruvate promotes weight loss. Because the substance has a critical role in the conversion of food to energy, proponents believe that Pyruvate supplements can improve fat utilization, increase the efficiency of energy production, and speed up the metabolism. Those who advocate its use as an endurance booster feel that it increases the supply of energy to the muscles.

An inability to process Pyruvate properly is at the root of several hereditary disorders. Defects in Pyruvate metabolism can lead to mental retardation, muscle and organ damage, or seizures. In times of physical stress, abnormalities in energy metabolism can lead to a dangerous buildup of lactic acid in the system (lactic acidosis).

Avoid if . . .
Do not take Pyruvate if you've been diagnosed with a disorder that affects its metabolism.

Special Cautions
Large doses of Pyruvate may cause gastrointestinal upset, including bloating, diarrhea, gas, gurgling sounds in the digestive tract, and upset stomach.

Commercial preparations of Pyruvate may contain extra ingredients such as sodium, potassium, magnesium, and calcium. If you have high blood pressure, suffer from a heart condition, or are taking any medications, check with your doctor before using a Pyruvate supplement.

Possible Drug Interactions
No interactions have been reported.

Special Information if You Are Pregnant or Breast-feeding
Pyruvate is not recommended for women who are pregnant or breast-feeding.

Available Preparations and Dosage
Pyruvate is available in capsule and powder form. Capsule strengths range from 500 to 1,000 milligrams of Pyruvate. Suppliers generally recommend dosages of 2 to 6 grams (2,000 to 6,000 milligrams) per day, taken in several small doses. If taken for weight loss, the supplement should not replace a comprehensive diet and exercise program.

Overdosage
No information on overdosage is available.

Red Yeast Rice

Why People Take It

Known in China as Hong-Qu, Red Yeast Rice is a standard part of the national cuisine—used, for example, in the preparation of Peking duck. For centuries, it has also been employed in traditional Chinese medicine to help maintain a healthy heart and circulatory system. Recent studies suggest there may be good reason. Research has shown that when taken along with a healthy low-cholesterol diet and regular exercise, Red Yeast Rice may reduce cholesterol levels in people with mild to moderately high cholesterol (although how much of the benefit stems from diet and exercise alone remains undetermined).

What It Is; How It Works

Red Yeast Rice *(Monascus purpureus)* is made, quite simply, by fermenting red yeast on rice. A special process is used to isolate a higher concentration of the natural ingredient mevinolin. This substance is similar to the "statin" drugs, such as Zocor, Pravachol, and Lipitor, that doctors prescribe for high cholesterol. Products containing mevinolin, however, can be purchased without a prescription as over-the-counter dietary supplements under names such as Cholestin.

Everyone's body needs a certain amount of cholesterol to function properly. The substance is found in cell membranes and helps the body make certain hormones. But if too much cholesterol gets into the system, it can accumulate as fatty deposits in the arteries, increasing the risk of heart disease. The liver produces about 80 percent of the cholesterol we need, with the other 20 percent coming from food sources. Red Yeast Rice (and "statin" drugs) block the action of an enzyme in the liver that triggers cholesterol production. Some researchers also speculate that the unsaturated fatty acids in Red Yeast Rice could contribute to its beneficial effects.

Avoid if . . .
In very high doses, the mevinolin in Red Yeast Rice has been known to damage the liver. Do not take it if you have liver disease, are in danger of developing it, or consume more than two alcoholic beverages a day.

Special Cautions
It's best to stop using Red Yeast Rice during a serious infection. Avoid it, too, after major surgery. If you develop any muscle pain or weakness, discontinue the product immediately and check with your doctor.

Possible Drug Interactions
Do not combine Red Yeast Rice with prescription cholesterol-lowering drugs, antifungal medications, drugs

that suppress the immune system, or erythromycin. These drugs may increase the chance of muscle pain and weakness.

Special Information if You Are Pregnant or Breast-feeding

Because generous supplies of cholesterol are needed by a developing baby, you should strictly avoid Red Yeast Rice during pregnancy. You should also avoid it while breast-feeding.

Available Preparations and Dosage

Red Yeast Rice is available commercially in capsule form. The typical dosage recommendation is 1,200 milligrams per day, divided into two doses. Do not exceed 2,400 milligrams daily. Take with food to reduce the risk of digestive disturbance.

Overdosage

In animal tests, massive overdoses of mevinolin produced no ill effects. Nevertheless, if you suspect a problem, be sure to check with your doctor.

Ribose

Why People Take It

A type of simple sugar, Ribose is taken by athletes in an effort to increase energy, endurance, alertness, and lean muscle mass, and to reduce fatigue and recovery time following exercise.

What It Is; How It Works

Ribose is one of the key constituents of the human body. Produced during digestion, it's one of the building blocks of DNA and RNA, the compounds that carry the genetic code and interpret its instructions for building proteins.

Ribose also is one of the main components of ATP (adenosine triphosphate), the compound that serves as the primary source of energy for all the cells in the body. In muscle cells, excess ATP molecules are joined with the chemical creatine to create a reserve form of fuel.

During exercise, the cells break down ATP to release its energy. ATP used up in this fashion is replaced by the body during the following hours and days, using Ribose and other chemicals as raw materials. The extra Ribose gained from supplements is supposed to speed up production of new ATP, hastening the return to normal levels.

Avoid if . . .
Do not take Ribose supplements if you have gout or diabetes.

Special Cautions
Use Ribose judiciously. Large doses may cause diarrhea, stomach upset, and low blood sugar.

Possible Drug Interactions
No interactions have been reported.

Special Information if You Are Pregnant or Breast-feeding
Harmful effects seem unlikely, and none are known. Nevertheless, as with any supplement that's not required for good health, the safest course is to avoid Ribose during pregnancy.

Available Preparations and Dosage
Ribose supplements are available in capsule, lozenge, tablet, powder, and syrup form. Some products are available in different flavors. Ribose is also an ingredient in some combination supplements that include creatine.

A single dose usually consists of 2 to 3 grams of Ribose. Suppliers often recommend that athletes take a divided dose, one part before a workout and one part after. Some suppliers also recommend a larger "loading dose" in certain situations.

Overdosage
No information on overdosage is available.

RNA (Ribonucleic Acid)

Why People Take It

A key component of every living cell, RNA (ribonucleic acid) is the compound that transmits the instructions coded into our DNA. As such, it has been the subject of a variety of exaggerated claims. For example, some proponents insist that supplemental RNA can slow aging and improve memory. They say it can enhance vision and hearing, create tighter, more radiant skin, and restore vitality and sexual vigor. Unfortunately, there's no evidence that it actually does any of these things.

What it *may* do is bolster the body's ability to ward off infection. A number of studies conducted on animals have demonstrated that a diet supplemented with RNA enhances immune response and helps restore lost immune function and maintain it. Moreover, clinical studies have found that critically ill and malnourished patients whose diets are supplemented with RNA often exhibit an improved immune response. Likewise, studies in cancer patients have shown that RNA supplementation seems to reduce the chance of infection and postoperative surgical complications. Some clinical trials also suggest that RNA supplementation can help maintain normal growth and development in infants.

Nevertheless, there's still a chance that these benefits stem from some other nutrient in a person's diet, so most experts regard the evidence as inconclusive. And whether or not the effects are genuine, the supplements seem to do no more than bring a weakened immune system up to par. They won't provide any extra boost to someone who's already fit.

What It Is; How It Works
Produced in the nucleus of each cell, RNA governs the construction of proteins from various combinations of amino acids. Both RNA and DNA are integral parts of all human cells—and of everything we eat.

Laboratory and animal studies suggest that RNA supplements improve the body's resistance by stimulating the proliferation of T lymphocytes and macrophages—two key players in the immune system's ongoing defense against invading germs and toxins.

Avoid if . . .
There are no reported reasons to avoid RNA supplements.

Special Cautions
Check with your doctor for a reliable source of RNA. Contaminated products could harbor infectious agents.

Possible Drug Interactions
No interactions have been reported.

Special Information if You Are Pregnant or Breast-feeding
The effect of RNA supplementation during pregnancy remains unknown. As with all supplements, your safest course is to avoid it while pregnant.

During breast-feeding, however, RNA might actually prove beneficial. Compounds containing RNA and DNA (nucleotides) are released naturally by the breakdown of cells in breast milk. In at least one study, infants who were fed breast milk or nucleotide-enriched formula showed greater macrophage activity than babies who were fed unsupplemented formula. Still, despite this apparent benefit, it's a good idea to consult your doctor before taking an RNA supplement.

Available Preparations and Dosage
RNA is typically used as an ingredient in combination dietary supplements. It can also be found in powder and tablet form, in strengths ranging from 25 to 250 milligrams. No recommended dietary allowance has been established.

Overdosage
No information on overdosage is available.

Royal Jelly

Why People Take It

Thanks to a striking disparity in the life spans of bees, Royal Jelly has enjoyed a long and undeserved reputation as an antiaging agent and purported aphrodisiac. Produced from the salivary glands of bees, it serves as food for both the bees' immature larvae and their queen. The ordinary larvae feed on it for only the first few days of life, then change into worker bees and, within six weeks, die. The queen, however, continues to consume Royal Jelly for the remainder of her fertile life—and, for the queen, life can last up to five years! Noting this tremendous discrepancy, seers in both medieval Europe and China adopted Royal Jelly as a cure for old age.

Modern science has failed to find any evidence that Royal Jelly actually extends life. However, it does have some other potentially beneficial effects. It seems to reduce cholesterol levels in humans and laboratory animals, and one German study found that it may also be helpful in reducing some of the symptoms of menopause. Several studies involving experimental animals suggest that it may strengthen the immune system and fight cancerous tumors. Laboratory tests show that it also has some antibacterial properties.

Enthusiasts offer an extensive list of conditions that Royal Jelly supposedly relieves; the roster includes rheumatoid arthritis, bone and joint disorders, multiple sclerosis, lupus, chronic fatigue syndrome, kidney and liver disease, pancreatitis, insomnia, headaches, stomach ulcers, and skin disorders. They also claim that Royal Jelly can increase energy and help support weight loss. There has been no research to date, however, that supports any of these assertions.

One claim made for Royal Jelly is not only baseless but potentially dangerous: Some proponents recommend it for asthma. There are many documented reports of respiratory distress, asthmatic attack, anaphylaxis (extreme allergic reaction), and even death among people who are allergic to bee products. For someone with allergies, asthma, or any other respiratory condition to even consider using Royal Jelly would therefore be foolhardy.

Royal Jelly's antiaging mystique has also brought it popularity as an additive in many skin-care products, including creams, lotions, soaps, and cosmetics. Manufacturers claim that some of the ingredients in Royal Jelly support collagen production and slow the effects of aging on skin, though there's no conclusive evidence of this.

What It Is; How It Works

Analysis of Royal Jelly shows it contains a rich blend of proteins, unsaturated fats, enzymes, sugar, all of the essential amino acids, and ample quantities of minerals and vitamins, especially the B vitamins and, in particular, pantothenic acid. Many of the current claims for Royal

Jelly seem to be based on the known health benefits of this complex mixture of ingredients. (There are, however, many other ways to get the same proteins, minerals, and vitamins without exposing yourself to the risks of Royal Jelly.)

The cancer-fighting compound in Royal Jelly has been tentatively identified as 10-HDA (10-hydroxy-2-decanoic acid), and 10-HDA levels are used as an index of the amount of Royal Jelly a product actually contains. Tests for 10-HDA reveal that the buyer definitely had better beware. They show that many products claiming to be pure Royal Jelly contain little of it—or none at all. (As dietary supplements, Royal Jelly products are subject to minimal inspection and regulation.)

Avoid if . . .

Do not take Royal Jelly if you are allergic to bee pollen or other bee products, have asthma, or suffer from any other respiratory condition. There are reports of respiratory distress, anaphylaxis, and death among susceptible people following ingestion of Royal Jelly products. People who tend to have allergies can be at risk even if they don't suffer from asthma.

Special Cautions

Royal Jelly products such as creams and lotions applied to the skin can cause skin inflammation in people who are sensitive to bee products.

Possible Drug Interactions

There are no known drug interactions with Royal Jelly.

Special Information if You Are Pregnant or Breast-feeding

Authentic Royal Jelly is a potpourri of chemicals, and its effects during pregnancy have not been carefully studied. Your best course is to avoid it while pregnant or breast-feeding.

Available Preparations and Dosage

Royal Jelly products come in tablets, capsules, gel caps, and ampules containing 50 to 500 milligrams. Manufacturers' dosage recommendations vary widely. Royal Jelly is also available in creams, lotions, and soaps for topical use according to package recommendations.

Overdosage

No information on overdosage is available.

SAMe (S-Adenosylmethionine)

Why People Take It

In a series of small but promising clinical trials, this over-the-counter remedy for depression has proved itself the equal of traditional prescription drugs. Though some authorities dismiss it as a mild mood-lifter, others regard it as an important new medication, since it has not only performed as well as potent "tricyclic" antidepressants, but it also starts working faster (within one or two weeks, versus three to four weeks or longer for standard drugs). Outside the United States, it has been sold for years as a prescription antidepressant, mainly under the name AdoMet.

SAMe has been studied as an aid to the effectiveness of other antidepressants, with promising results. It also has been found to provide at least some relief from postpartum depression and depression associated with Parkinson's disease and epilepsy. In addition, it has been tested for usefulness against a number of other neurological disorders, including schizophrenia, Alzheimer's disease, and dementia. Although these tests are far from conclusive, they've produced encouraging results.

SAMe is also used to treat osteoarthritis, the type of arthritis caused by wear and tear on the protective cartilage in the joints. Preliminary studies appear to confirm its ability to relieve stiffness, pain, and swelling. However, there's no evidence to support manufacturers' claims that it can renew damaged cartilage. SAMe also shows promise as a treatment for the painful muscle condition called fibromyalgia. And studies show that supplementation with SAMe can improve liver function, making it a candidate for treatment of cirrhosis, impaired bile flow, and liver damage from drugs or alcohol.

Claims that SAMe is useful in the treatment of heart disease and cancer are currently unsubstantiated, though preliminary clinical studies are under way. Assertions that SAMe fights the effects of aging also remain unproven.

What It Is; How It Works

SAMe is a natural substance found in the body's cells. The body manufactures it from the essential amino acid methionine. In turn, it plays an important role in the production of a wide variety of hormones, amino acids, antioxidants, and chemical messengers in the brain. Researchers have noted low levels of SAMe in people with depression, and have found that SAMe rises as depression improves. SAMe also helps maintain the strength and flexibility of cell walls, and it participates in the production of DNA and RNA.

SAMe supplements are especially helpful in cases of liver disease, which depletes the body's natural supply. Extra vitamins B_6, B_{12}, and folic acid are usually recommended with SAMe supplementation. In fact, some products already have them added.

When purchasing a SAMe product, be sure to ask for a reliable brand. Independent analyses of SAMe products have found that the content varies widely, with at least one brand containing almost no usable SAMe. About half the brands tested delivered all that they claimed.

Avoid if . . .

It's best to avoid SAMe if you have bipolar disorder (manic-depressive illness); it can cause episodes of mania. People taking antidepressants should not discontinue their medication or start taking SAMe without their physician's advice.

Special Cautions

If you're already taking a prescription antidepressant, check with your doctor before attempting to replace it with SAMe or add SAMe to your regimen. You may need to reduce your dose gradually.

If you suffer from high homocysteine levels (a condition associated with increased risk of heart disease), you might want to consider adding the homocysteine-lowering supplement TMG to your regimen (see separate entry). Homocysteine is a by-product of SAMe.

Unlike some prescription antidepressants, SAMe is said to have no serious side effects. However, some people suffer mild attacks of indigestion, anxiety, insomnia, mania, and hyperactive muscles.

Possible Drug Interactions
SAMe may reduce the effectiveness of some medications, including the Parkinson's disease medication L-dopa.

Special Information if You Are Pregnant or Breast-feeding
The safety of SAMe supplements during pregnancy has not been determined. Check with your doctor before using SAMe while pregnant or breast-feeding.

Available Preparations and Dosage
Synthetic SAMe is available in tablets, usually in strengths of 200 or 400 milligrams. For depression, some authorities recommend dosages of 400 to 1,600 milligrams per day. For arthritis, recommendations vary from 200 to 1,200 milligrams per day. For liver disease, daily dosages of 1,600 milligrams are common. The daily total is divided into smaller doses. They should be taken 1 hour before or 2 hours after meals.

Some forms of SAMe tend to degrade quickly at any

temperature above freezing. Look for a temperature-stable form in a coated tablet. Store away from moisture.

Overdosage

No information on overdosage is available.

Soy Isoflavones

Why People Take Them

Soy has enjoyed a sudden surge of popularity in this country, largely thanks to the estrogenlike compounds known as Soy Isoflavones. For postmenopausal women, these compounds have offered the hope of estrogen's benefits without its accompanying risks—in particular the risk of breast cancer. Unfortunately, while soy-based *foods* offer well-documented health benefits, the jury is still out on refined Soy Isoflavone *supplements*.

Numerous studies show that Asian women, whose diets tend to be high in soy, have lower rates of breast, ovarian, and uterine cancers than do women who eat a typical American diet. And certain lab tests show that isoflavones can inhibit the growth of cancerous cells. However, other research in animals and humans suggest that Soy Isoflavones may *increase* cancer risk by stimulating breast cell growth.

Timing could be the secret behind this Jekyll-and-Hyde quality: Some scientists speculate that eating soy early in life, as many Asian women do, may protect against breast cancer, while not eating it until later in life may promote cancer in susceptible individuals. Dosage could also be involved: the modest amounts of isoflavones found in food may be protective, while the high doses provided by isoflavone supplements may have the opposite effect. At this point, the only thing that can be said with certainty is that we simply don't know whether the isoflavones in soy can help or hinder cancer.

And so it goes with the isoflavones' other potential benefits. Many advocates have recommended them for menopausal hot flashes, but a recent study designed to test their effectiveness for this purpose found that isoflavone supplements worked no better than an inactive pill. Evidence hints that a soy-rich diet may reduce the risk of prostate cancer and help protect against osteoporosis, but researchers don't know whether isoflavones are the ingredients responsible. Likewise, soy protein's indisputable effect on high cholesterol levels may or may not be due to the isoflavones it contains.

The reason we know so little about isoflavones is that most of the research on soy has centered on food products, not supplements. Scientists note that a whole food behaves differently in the body than a single compound. There could be numerous protective components in soy besides isoflavones. And because the isoflavone content in pills tends to be much higher than that in natural foods, the potential risks could be greater as well—particularly for women who have estrogen-dependent breast cancer.

That's why, at least for now, most researchers recommend avoiding isoflavone supplements.

What They Are; How They Work

Isoflavones belong to a group of plant chemicals known as phytoestrogens (see separate entry). The most-researched Soy Isoflavones are genistein, daidzein, and glycitein. Scientists are still unraveling how they work, but they seem to compete with human estrogen by attaching to hormone receptors in the body. In theory, this can produce a moderating effect. If there's too little estrogen in the body, isoflavones may attach to estrogen receptors and make up for the shortage. But if there's too much, isoflavones may "crowd out" some of the more potent human estrogen and keep it from activating hormonal receptors. Advocates believe this double-barreled action is what makes soy beneficial for both treating hot flashes (by increasing estrogen levels) and preventing cancer (by decreasing estrogen activity). Whether this is true remains to be verified.

Other research shows that isoflavones may have benefits unrelated to their estrogenlike effects. Some researchers believe that isoflavones could protect against cancer by promoting or inhibiting certain enzymes that affect tumor growth. Others say that they seem to work like antioxidants, neutralizing the highly reactive molecules, called free radicals, that can damage tissue when they get out of control.

Avoid if . . .

Women with hormone-dependent cancers, including breast, ovarian, and uterine cancers, should not take isoflavone supplements. It is also best to avoid the supplements if you have a family history of these diseases.

Special Cautions

Although soy foods pose no known health risks—and may even protect against cancer—women with hormone-dependent cancers should still check with their doctor before adding soy to their diet.

Possible Drug Interactions

It is not known whether Soy Isoflavones interact with medications. If you take any medicine on a regular basis, check with your doctor before taking this supplement.

Special Information if You Are Pregnant or Breast-feeding

Because of the isoflavones' estrogenlike activity, women who are pregnant or breast-feeding should avoid isoflavone supplements.

Available Preparations and Dosage

Supplements are available in tablet, capsule, liquid, and powder form. Products should contain a mixture of isoflavones, including genistein and daidzein. Manufacturers recommend taking isoflavone supplements with a large glass of warm water at mealtime. Also be aware that a high-fiber meal may interfere with their absorption.

Manufacturers' dosage recommendations for hot flashes range from 200 to 600 milligrams a day. For prostate problems, a typical dosage recommendation is 1,000 milligrams of a standardized supplement containing 5 percent isoflavones.

If you choose to boost your intake of soy products instead of taking supplements, remember that the isoflavone content of soy foods varies widely, depending on the plant species, growing conditions, and how the soybeans are processed, among other things. For example, one-half cup of roasted soybeans can contain as much as 170 milligrams of isoflavones, while one cup of soy milk generally has only 20 to 50 milligrams. The typical soy-rich diet in Japan provides 25 to 50 milligrams of isoflavones a day.

Overdosage
No information on overdosage is available.

Soy Protein

Why People Take It
The U.S. Food and Drug Administration allows only a handful of foods to carry specific health claims on their labels, and Soy Protein is one of them. In October 1999, government researchers agreed that eating 25 grams of Soy Protein a day can lower your cholesterol levels and thereby reduce the risk of heart disease. To get these benefits, however, remember that you must also follow a diet low in saturated fat and cholesterol.

The FDA approved this health claim after research

showed that a daily intake of at least 25 grams of Soy Protein could lower LDL, or "bad," cholesterol by up to 10 percent, a reduction that's known to cut the risk of heart disease in people with a severe cholesterol problem. Other research has found that Soy Protein can also lower blood pressure and total cholesterol levels. And some experts suggest that because Soy Protein is easier for the kidneys to process than animal protein, it may play a useful role in the treatment of kidney problems resulting from diabetes and other diseases.

Some evidence suggests that soy, in addition to fostering a healthy heart, may be helpful for treating such illnesses as menopausal hot flashes, osteoporosis, and even certain cancers. Many advocates, however, feel that these potential benefits are due to soy isoflavones (see separate entry), not Soy Protein per se. Isoflavones extracted from soy exhibit significantly different properties than those of ordinary Soy Protein—and some researchers fear they may even pose cancer risks. According to the FDA, however, these issues do not apply to whole foods such as tofu or soy milk, or to intact Soy Protein added to other foods.

What It Is; How It Works

The protein in soy is "complete"—that is, it contains all 20 of the amino acids needed for human health. And soybeans are the only vegetable source of protein that is comparable to the protein in animal foods.

How Soy Protein lowers cholesterol and other blood fats is unclear. Researchers speculate that by eating more soy, you'll eat fewer animal foods, which are relatively high in saturated fat and cholesterol. Others suggest that soy may alter hormonal levels, which in turn signals the liver to make less cholesterol. In addition, many soy products are rich in fiber, which has been shown to reduce cholesterol and other blood fats.

Avoid if . . .

There are no known risks in eating the Soy Protein that occurs naturally in whole foods. But women with hormone-dependent cancers (such as breast, ovarian, and uterine cancers) should discuss with their doctor whether to avoid soy-based extracts and supplements, due to the possible presence of isoflavones. It may also be best to avoid such products if you have a family history of these diseases.

Special Cautions

Soy Protein allergies, although rare, are possible. Studies estimate that 0.5 percent of children, and even fewer adults, are allergic to soy. Raw, unprocessed soy foods are generally more likely to cause allergic reactions than roasted soybeans or those foods that undergo chemical or heat processing (tofu, for example).

Possible Drug Interactions

No interactions are known.

Special Information if You Are Pregnant or Breast-feeding

Because of the isoflavone content in certain soy-based supplements, women who are pregnant or breast-feeding should not take them. Whole soy foods, however, are considered safe.

Available Preparations and Dosage

According to the FDA, a product must provide at least 25 grams of Soy Protein a day (typically in four 6.25-gram portions) to improve cholesterol levels. Remember too that the emphasis is on *daily* Soy Protein intake; you can't just have it once in a while.

Supplements containing Soy Protein usually use soybeans that have been processed by heat or chemical treatments. These include soy protein concentrate, soy protein isolates, textured soy protein, and meat substitutes made with Soy Protein. A variety of supplements are available in powder forms, drink mixes, and "energy" bars. Soy Protein is also found in many of the products used by bodybuilders and athletes. When using the supplements, follow the manufacturer's recommendations.

Be aware that some Soy Protein products could contain flavorings such as monosodium glutamate (MSG), an additive often found in Chinese food that causes adverse reactions in some people. Another caveat: Soy protein isolates that are processed using alcohol extraction (rather than water extraction) have significantly lower levels of potentially beneficial isoflavones. In contrast, soy protein isolates in general have the highest protein content of all Soy Protein products.

Overdosage

No information on overdosage is available.

Spirulina

Why People Take It

It's amazing but true: The maestros of health and fitness have succeeded in taking a foul-tasting pond scum, promoting it as a cure-all "superfood," and selling tons of it. Spirulina, a form of blue-green algae, actually does have an unusual concentration—and combination—of nutrients. There's also a possibility that it may eventually prove to have certain antiviral and anticancer properties. However, all of the nutrients it offers are easily obtained—at far lower cost—in conventional foods. Its therapeutic effects have yet to be scientifically demonstrated. And its purported abilities to "detoxify," "boost energy," or help weight loss are all without foundation.

What It Is; How it Works

Spirulina, a substance composed of microscopic freshwater plants, is harvested commercially in huge manmade ponds, dried, and sold as pills or powder. Promoters point out that it is packed with protein, beta-carotene, vitamin B_{12}, and gamma-linolenic acid (GLA). Legitimate nutrition experts confirm this, but point out that there's scant reason to obtain any of these nutrients from an expensive, exotic source like Spirulina when they are readily available elsewhere.

In general, the health claims made for Spirulina are wildly exaggerated. It's true, for instance, that cultivation of blue-green algae has been eyed as an alternative protein source in impoverished countries, and that the World Health Organization (WHO) used Spirulina to help feed protein-deficient children in India. But most Americans eat too much protein, not too little, and can get high-quality protein from lean meat and eggs for a fraction of the cost of Spirulina.

Similarly, the WHO found that 1 gram of Spirulina daily reduced the incidence of Bitot's spots (a type of blindness caused by vitamin A deficiency) by supplying victims with adequate amounts of the vitamin A precursor beta-carotene. But beta-carotene can be obtained in abundance from a variety of inexpensive fruits and vegetables.

It's also a fact that Spirulina is packed with vitamin B_{12} (found mainly in animal products), but it is a form of B_{12} that the human body can't use. And one species of Spirulina does indeed contain high levels of gamma-linolenic acid, an essential fatty acid with anti-inflammatory effects. However, supplement labels are not required to list which species is contained in the product, and there are over a thousand species.

As promised, blue-green algae products also contain an array of nutrients and phytochemicals that are being tested for protective effects against cancer, viruses, and other conditions, either alone, in combination, or in the form of extracts. But the jury is still out on the value of

these substances, and Spirulina itself has not been scientifically proven to offer immune support or cure any disease.

Finally, Spirulina has been touted as a safe, natural
weight-loss aid because it contains the amino acid phenylalanine, which supposedly acts as an appetite suppressant (see separate entry). However, the U.S. Food and
Drug Administration has debunked these claims, con-
cluding that there is no evidence that phenylalanine—or
Spirulina—reduces the appetite.

Avoid if . . .
There have been a few reports of allergy to blue-green
algae. If you have a history of food allergies, use the
product with caution. Large amounts of Spirulina, which
are high in protein, would also be inappropriate for
anyone who is on a protein-restricted diet for medical
reasons (such as kidney failure).

Special Cautions
No side effects are associated with Spirulina or other
blue-green algae, but concerns have been raised over the
purity of these supplements. Liver toxins were found in
another type of blue-green algae (not Spirulina, but concern persists over the actual type and content of algae in
Spirulina supplements).

Possible Drug Interactions
There are no reported drug interactions with Spirulina.

Special Information if You Are Pregnant or Breast-feeding
There's no evidence that Spirulina is harmful during
pregnancy. But since it hasn't been formally tested for

safety, and since you can easily find alternative sources for the nutrients it supplies, your safest course is to avoid it while pregnant or breast-feeding.

Available Preparations and Dosage

Spirulina is available in 30- to 100-milligram capsules and tablets from a number of leading supplement manufacturers, and can also be taken in bulk or powdered form. Manufacturers typically recommend a total daily intake of 2 to 3 grams (2,000 to 3,000 milligrams), taken in several small doses.

Overdosage

There is no well-established threshold for an overdosage of Spirulina. Its chief "active ingredients" are not associated with significant risk of overdose in the quantities you're likely to obtain from it.

Streptococcus Thermophilus

Why People Take It

Despite its forbidding name, *Streptococcus thermophilus* is actually a beneficial type of microorganism that protects the body from the germs that cause diarrhea. Known as probiotics, these friendly bacteria reside in the lower intestine, rendering it uninhabitable for a variety of their less beneficial cousins, as well as the fungus responsible for yeast infections. Some evidence suggests that these beneficial bacteria may also improve cholesterol profiles and protect against certain cancers.

What It Is; How It Works

Streptococcus thermophilus is one of the two types of bacteria most often used to produce cultured dairy foods such as cheese, sour cream, and yogurt. (The other is lactobacillus; see separate entry.) When you eat yogurt containing live cultures, you ingest millions of these friendly bacteria. Although up to 90 percent die on their way to the lower intestine, enough survive to make the environment uncomfortable for disease-causing bacteria. They do this by breaking down lactose (milk sugar) into lactic acid, which increases the overall acidity of the intestine enough to kill off large numbers of harmful germs, including those that cause botulism, salmonellosis, diarrhea, and yeast infections.

Some researchers believe that *Streptococcus thermophilus* may also play a role in controlling cholesterol levels. There are at least two ways in which these bacteria could accomplish this. As the bacteria in the lower intestine ferment, they produce compounds called short-chain fatty acids (SCFAs). One SCFA—propionic acid—has been shown to decrease cholesterol production in the liver, thus reducing the amount of cholesterol circulating in the blood. Some bacteria also have the ability to break down the cholesterol-rich bile acids that the liver pours into the intestines. These acids are largely reabsorbed, so that most of their cholesterol is recycled back into the body. But if the bile acids are broken down, their cholesterol is flushed out as waste instead of returning to the bloodstream.

There are also theories that probiotic bacteria may help fend off certain types of cancer. Many of these bacteria produce volatile fatty acids that have been shown to inhibit the growth of certain cancer cells. Some researchers suggest that the bacteria may also contain or produce enzymes that detoxify potential cancer-causing agents as they pass through the intestine.

Streptococcus thermophilus supplements are totally unnecessary as long as your native population of probiotic bacteria is sufficient to maintain their health. However, antibiotics, chronic diarrhea, and poor eating habits often serve to give harmful bacteria the upper hand. High-fat, high-sugar diets encourage proliferation of undesirable organisms, while emotional stress seems to lower the count of friendly ones. If you face any one of these problems, extra probiotics might prove beneficial.

Avoid if . . .
There is no known reason to avoid *Streptococcus thermophilus*.

Special Cautions
Because probiotic supplements contain living organisms, freshness is important. Purchase the supplements well before their expiration date. Once the supplements are opened, refrigerate them, and throw them out when they are more than six months old. At that point, the organisms are dead.

Possible Drug Interactions
No interactions are known.

Special Information if You Are Pregnant or Breast-feeding
No specific information is available. However, it's wise to check with your doctor before taking any supplement while pregnant or breast-feeding.

Available Preparations and Dosage
Streptococcus thermophilus can be obtained from certain yogurts. Check the label to make sure you're purchasing a brand that contains live cultures. *Streptococcus thermophilus* is also found in certain probiotic supplemental preparations, usually available in the form of capsules, powders, or liquids.

Follow the manufacturer's directions for supplement dosage. Most experts advise against taking probiotics continuously. Instead, they recommend reserving them for short courses to repopulate the colon with friendly flora after antibiotic therapy, to treat intestinal yeast overgrowth, or to stave off infectious diarrhea when traveling in underdeveloped countries.

Overdosage
No information on overdosage is available.

Sulforaphane

Why People Take It

Sulforaphane is a member of the intriguing new class of nutritional compounds known as phytochemicals. Found in plant-based foods, including fruits, vegetables, and grains, a number of these organic chemicals have shown signs of exciting health-enhancing properties. Scientists already know that Mother Nature uses phytochemicals to protect plants against bugs and too much sun. Now they're finding that some of them, including Sulforaphane, may also serve as potent inhibitors of cancer and other diseases.

Sulforaphane is abundant in cruciferous vegetables like broccoli and cauliflower. A few years ago, researchers discovered they could easily extract Sulforaphane from broccoli sprouts. When they gave it to laboratory animals, the compound lowered the rate of breast cancer, and also reduced the size of tumors that did develop. On further study, they realized that certain strains of the sprouts contained up to 100 times more Sulforaphane than mature broccoli florets. A trial designed to study the effects of these supercharged broccoli sprouts in humans is now under way.

Other studies hint that Sulforaphane may also lower

the risk of bladder and colon cancer. But though the early findings are promising, more investigation is needed before we can be sure. For instance, the study on colon cancer was conducted, not in humans, but on cultured cells in the lab. And although the one on bladder cancer verified that a diet high in cruciferous vegetables (especially broccoli and cabbage) is associated with a lower risk of the disease, purified Sulforaphane alone wasn't given a test.

Nevertheless, many supplement manufacturers are now including Sulforaphane in their products. Their rationale? Because a lot of us fail to eat the recommended servings of vegetables—and some of us wouldn't touch broccoli if our lives depended on it—taking Sulforaphane in pill form is supposed to act as a kind of insurance policy for our health.

What It Is; How It Works

Sulforaphane spurs the production of natural detoxifying enzymes in the body. In the case of breast cancer, the compound seems to make certain enzymes in breast cells jump into action, locating potentially cancer-causing substances and locking those substances to molecules that remove them from the cells. However, scientists still don't know exactly how much Sulforaphane is needed to trigger this search-and-destroy mission, or whether it performs better in concert with other nutrients.

Many nutritionists caution that, although it sounds attractive to distill the benefits of certain vegetables and put them in a pill, it's probably an *array* of phytochemicals from a wide variety of plants that provides the maximum benefit. No single phytochemical, they say, is likely to be the silver bullet against cancer. Until all the results are in, they still recommend eating a variety of vegetables—including the cruciferous ones—to provide your body with a full set of tools for fighting off cancer and other diseases.

There is one way to radically boost your Sulforaphane intake without relying on supplements: eat plenty of broccoli sprouts. Researchers at Johns Hopkins University have developed a strain that contains from 30 to 50 times more Sulforaphane than the average head of mature broccoli. Eating a half cup of these designer sprouts—sold in stores as BroccoSprouts—is equal to eating three and one-half cups of the cooked mature vegetable. Unlike other "enhanced" foods, these mildly spicy sprouts are in no way genetically altered—they're merely younger versions of the full-grown plant.

Avoid if . . .
Because no long-term safety studies have been conducted with human subjects, it is not known whether certain people should avoid taking Sulforaphane in supplement form. So far, animal and lab tests have yet to uncover any significant side effects.

Special Cautions
While the reasons to increase your intake of Sulforaphane sound compelling, scientists point out that many chemicals found to protect against cancer in animal studies or laboratory tests have failed to have the same effect in humans.

Possible Drug Interactions

It is not known whether Sulforaphane supplements interact with any medications.

Special Information if You Are Pregnant or Breast-feeding

The effects of taking extra Sulforaphane during pregnancy and breast-feeding are unknown. As with any supplement or medication, it's best to avoid using it during this period unless absolutely necessary. You can get plenty of Sulforaphane from vegetables.

Available Preparations and Dosage

Sulforaphane is available in capsule and powder form. Dosage recommendations vary according to the manufacturer. Some manufacturers claim that one capsule of Sulforaphane equals one serving of cruciferous vegetables, usually broccoli. Others say that one capsule is equivalent to 1 pound, or close to 2 servings. Sulforaphane can also be found in comprehensive supplements containing a variety of phytochemicals. It is often listed as "broccoli extract."

If you choose to augment your diet with specially grown, Sulforaphane-rich broccoli sprouts, the suggested intake is two or three half-cup servings a week. You can find the sprouts in the produce section of many supermarkets.

Overdosage

No information on overdosage is available.

Taurine

Why People Take It

This common amino acid was largely ignored by medical researchers until the early 1970s, when serious investigations first began. To date, it has shown its greatest promise as a supplemental treatment for congestive heart failure (CHF) and epilepsy.

Taurine is an accepted treatment for CHF in Japan, and several U.S. studies have confirmed its benefits. In one double-blind trial (in which neither the patients nor their doctors knew who was receiving actual Taurine), 58 people with CHF showed improvement in several measures while taking 2 grams of Taurine 3 times daily for 4 weeks. A second double-blind study was also encouraging.

Studies of Taurine's use in treating epilepsy have been less conclusive, with researchers calling for more, better-controlled trials in this area. Some studies have found that Taurine may also be beneficial for cystic fibrosis patients who have difficulty absorbing nutrients. Other studies have suggested that it may be helpful in lowering cholesterol, as well as in treating some eye diseases, liver diseases, and diabetes. Although experts say these results are promising, they assert that more research is needed before the product can be widely recommended for any of these conditions.

Some proponents of Taurine suspect that it might be useful in the treatment of Alzheimer's disease. However, there have been no significant trials to date.

What It Is; How It Works

Taurine is best known as a component of the liver's bile acids, used by the body to help absorb fats and fat-soluble vitamins. But it also plays many other important roles in metabolism, especially in the nervous system and muscles. High levels of Taurine are found in the heart, the brain, and the retina of the eye, as well as in white blood cells. Taurine helps regulate the heartbeat, affects the release of the nervous system's chemical messengers, and maintains cell membranes.

Taurine is considered a "nonessential" amino acid, since the body can produce its own supply when there's a shortage in the diet. The body manufactures it from vitamin B_6 and the amino acids methionine and cysteine. Taurine also is readily available from foods such as eggs, fish, meat, and milk. Only infants do not make enough of it to meet their needs, although the amounts supplied by breast milk or infant formula are sufficient to make up the difference. Adults—even strict vegetarians—do not need supplemental Taurine to maintain good health.

Avoid if . . .

Don't take Taurine if you are allergic to proteins such as those in eggs, milk, or wheat.

Special Cautions

If you have a serious medical condition such as congestive heart failure or epilepsy, don't try to treat yourself
with Taurine without seeing a doctor. You'll need other
medications, and your condition should be monitored by
a professional.

Possible Drug Interactions

Taurine tends to boost the effect of anticonvulsant medications, reducing the frequency of seizures. But before
adding it to your treatment regimen, check with your
doctor; dosages should be carefully monitored.

Special Information if You Are Pregnant or Breast-feeding

No specific information is available, but it's wise to
avoid any supplement during these periods unless it is
absolutely necessary.

Available Preparations and Dosage

Both tablets and capsules are available, in 500- and
1000-milligram strengths. Taurine is also included in a
number of combination preparations.

No official recommended dietary allowance has been established for Taurine, and there are no standard dosages.
A typical recommendation for epilepsy is 500 milligrams
3 times a day. For congestive heart failure, researchers have
used 2,000 milligrams 3 times daily.

Overdosage

Taurine is considered unlikely to cause serious symptoms, but high dosages may produce diarrhea and peptic
ulcers.

TMG (Trimethylglycine)

Why People Take It

TMG's sudden popularity stems from its ability to reduce blood levels of homocysteine, an amino acid compound that has been linked to heart disease. At normal levels, your body uses homocysteine to manufacture other amino acids. But research shows that people with high blood levels of this substance have an increased risk for heart problems and blood-vessel damage.

Two small trials in people with abnormally high homocysteine levels confirmed that TMG can eliminate excess quantities of this compound. One study was conducted among people whose levels remained high despite treatment with vitamin B_6 and folate—a common therapy for high homocysteine. Adding TMG to the regimen brought their levels close to normal. The other study verified TMG's ability to maintain reduced homocysteine levels for up to 13 years. The authors pointed out that the benefit soon disappeared after the supplements were stopped.

A few studies hint that homocysteine may also be a risk factor for other diseases—depression, diabetes, stroke, liver disease, and Alzheimer's disease, among others.

Whether TMG supplementation would be helpful for these conditions remains largely unexplored. However, an animal-based study did show that TMG protected against the early stages of liver injury due to alcoholism, although the findings have yet to be duplicated in humans.

Because of homocysteine's link with hardening of the arteries and heart disease, finding ways to lower it has been a goal of much ongoing research. Scientists already know that certain B vitamins, particularly B_6 and folate, can help keep homocysteine from accumulating in the blood. They've also confirmed, in a Harvard University study of over 80,000 nurses, that taking supplements of these vitamins is in fact associated with a reduced risk of heart attack. To date there's been no comparable trial of TMG, but it is not unreasonable to expect a similar benefit.

What It Is; How It Works

TMG (also called betaine) rids the blood of excess homocysteine by converting it to the amino acid methionine in a natural chemical reaction known as methylation. Methionine, in turn, serves as raw material for a variety of additional amino acids and other beneficial compounds, including S-adenosylmethionine, or SAMe, a natural substance that has been shown to fight depression (see separate entry). TMG's promoters credit this double-barreled action—decrease in homocysteine and increase in SAMe—for its therapeutic effects.

TMG occurs naturally in various foods; the best sources are beets and broccoli. In fact, most of the supplements are derived from beet sugars.

Avoid if . . .

Although very few long-term safety studies have been conducted, lab tests and limited human studies performed to date suggest that TMG is relatively safe.

Special Cautions

If your homocysteine levels are normal, you won't benefit from TMG. Only those with abnormally high homocysteine levels face the increased risk of heart disease that TMG *may* reduce. If you're concerned about your risk for heart disease, check with your doctor. A simple blood test can document whether your homocysteine levels are too high. Although there are no formal recommendations for homocysteine testing, people who might benefit include those with a family history of atherosclerosis (clogged arteries) and those who have heart problems but no known risk factors such as high blood pressure or cholesterol.

There are no studies documenting the side effects of TMG. Proponents say that taking large amounts of the supplement without food can cause tension headaches.

Possible Drug Interactions

It is not known whether TMG interacts with medications. If you take any medicine on a regular basis, check with your doctor before taking this supplement.

Special Information if You Are Pregnant or Breast-feeding

TMG's safety during pregnancy has not been evaluated, and a temporary interruption in treatment is unlikely to affect your long-term health. Therefore your wisest course is to avoid TMG while pregnant or breast-feeding.

Available Preparations and Dosage

TMG is also known chemically as glycine betaine. If you're buying a supplement, be sure to get this kind of betaine. Another version called betaine hydrochloride (betaine HCl) does *not* lower homocysteine and may increase stomach acid.

TMG is available in tablet and powder form. The powder must be mixed with liquid, such as water or juice. For maximum effectiveness, manufacturers recommend taking TMG with food, along with vitamins B_6, B_{12}, and folate.

To lower homocysteine levels, suggested dosages range from 500 to 4,000 milligrams a day. For depression or liver problems, one manufacturer recommends taking 3,000 to 6,000 milligrams a day under the supervision of your doctor.

Overdosage

No information on overdosage is available.

Tryptophan

Why People Take It

In the 1980s, Tryptophan enjoyed widespread popularity as an inexpensive over-the-counter alternative to prescription antidepressants and sleep aids. Although research on the substance always produced mixed results, it was frequently recommended for depression, insomnia, and pain. It was used in the treatment of alcohol and cocaine addictions, and as a diet aid. Proponents claimed it could also be used for migraine headaches, premenstrual syndrome (PMS), obsessive-compulsive disorder, Alzheimer's disease, attention deficit disorder (ADD), autism, Parkinson's disease, and multiple sclerosis, among others.

Then in 1989 disaster struck. More than 1,500 people taking Tryptophan came down with a serious blood disease called eosinophilia-myalgia syndrome (EMS), and at least 30 people died of it. The U.S. Food and Drug Administration recalled all Tryptophan supplements from the market, and in 1990 it banned any further sales.

Most nutritional experts agree that the EMS outbreak was the result of contamination introduced by a single Japanese manufacturer of the substance. Nevertheless, over-the-counter Tryptophan supplements remain banned in the United States, though the substance is still added to infant formulas and intravenous feeding solutions, and can be obtained by prescription from a few special "compounding" pharmacies.

In its place, a related substance called 5-HTP (5-hydroxy-L-tryptophan) is now marketed in the United States for the same purposes as Tryptophan, although it's not clear that it works in exactly the same way. Caution is in order, however. In 1998, the FDA reported that the same contaminant that forced Tryptophan off the market in 1989 had been found in 5-HTP. Although the newer supplement hasn't been banned, the FDA has asked health professionals to report any illnesses associated with its use. Because of the risks involved, it's advisable to have your doctor monitor you if you decide to take 5-HTP.

What It Is; How It Works

Tryptophan is far from exotic. In fact, it is one of the eight essential amino acids that must be included in every diet because they can't be manufactured by the body. Like other amino acids, it's a building block of protein (although the body uses less of it than of the others). It's also necessary for the production of vitamin B_3 (niacin).

Any reasonable diet provides enough Tryptophan to meet the body's needs. Good sources include meat, fish, turkey, milk, cheese, eggs, fruits, nuts, and dates. Vitamin B_6 is required for its proper utilization. A lack of Tryptophan in the diet, like a shortage of protein in general, is thought to slow growth in children, cause apathy and weakness, and lead to a loss of hair color, weight loss, liver damage, and skin problems.

Tryptophan's reported therapeutic effects arise from its status as the raw material for serotonin. One of the nervous system's major chemical messengers, serotonin exerts a mood-lifting and calming effect on the brain. It also appears to play a role in pain control, and may reduce inflammation and stimulate movement in the digestive tract.

Research has confirmed that Tryptophan supplements produce an increase in serotonin levels. 5-HTP, which is formed from Tryptophan as an intermediate step in the production of serotonin, has a similar effect. Small trials of 5-HTP for anxiety and migraine have yielded definite, though moderate, improvement.

Avoid if . . .

Because Tryptophan supplements are banned in the United States, it's unwise to take any product labeled Tryptophan, L-tryptophan, Pacitron, Trofan, Tryptacin, or any other brand name for natural or synthetic Tryptophan. These products have not been checked for purity or safety, and therefore could lead to the potentially fatal blood disorder EMS.

Also avoid Tryptophan supplements—even by prescription—if you have asthma or lupus. Steer clear of 5-HTP if you have a digestive ailment such as an ulcer or Crohn's disease, or suffer from a rare condition called carcinoid syndrome that is associated with excessively high levels of serotonin in the blood.

Special Cautions

Tryptophan per se has only occasional mild side effects, such as nausea, headaches, and constipation. However, if you're unlucky enough to contract EMS from a contaminated supplement, you can expect symptoms such as high fever, muscle and joint pain, weakness, skin rash, and swelling of the arms and legs.

The most common side effects associated with 5-HTP are nausea and diarrhea. Occasionally, some people suffer grogginess.

Possible Drug Interactions

Tryptophan (and 5-HTP) may interact with prescription antidepressants, including monoamine oxidase inhibitors (MAO inhibitors). Check with your doctor before combining either supplement with such medications.

Special Information if You Are Pregnant or Breast-feeding
Do not take Tryptophan or related substances if you are
pregnant or breast-feeding.

Available Preparations and Dosage
Advocates of 5-HTP, the only substance related to tryptophan available on the U.S. market, often recommend
doses of 100 to 300 milligrams three times daily. In
clinical studies, it has been used in dosages ranging from
50 milligrams to 1,200 milligrams per day. It may take 2
or 3 weeks for antidepressant effects to appear.

Overdosage
High doses of 5-HTP can cause nausea and vomiting.

Tyrosine

Why People Take It
Tyrosine is the raw material for three of the nervous
system's leading chemical messengers: dopamine, norepinephrine, and epinephrine. Called neurotransmitters,
these substances pass messages from one nerve cell to the
next, helping to regulate brain function, muscle function,
body movement, and more.
    Deficiencies of these neurotransmitters can lead to

physical and mental fatigue and depression. Since all three are manufactured from Tyrosine, many people believe that boosting the supply of this substance can fight depression. Tyrosine has also been tried, without much success, in the treatment of attention deficit disorder (ADD) in children.

Studies have shown that Tyrosine may improve memory and alertness, and a limited military study indicates it may improve the ability to perform under stress. Other claims for Tyrosine remain unsubstantiated. They include assertions that it can improve sexual interest, relieve pain, and promote weight loss. Also, since dopamine is used to treat Parkinson's disease, Tyrosine has been proposed as a natural remedy for this movement disorder. It has been tried as a treatment for symptoms of alcohol withdrawal as well.

Athletes and bodybuilders take Tyrosine, most often in combination with other amino acids, but there is no evidence that Tyrosine itself helps to build muscles or improve endurance.

What It Is; How It Works

Tyrosine is one of the "nonessential" amino acids that the body can produce for itself. It's built from the amino acid phenylalanine with the help of vitamin B_6 and folic acid. Tyrosine is also abundant in meat, bananas, and papaya, and can be found in dairy products, oats, nuts, and fish. Although outright deficiencies of Tyrosine are rare, they are known to occur in people with kidney disease and in individuals who are unable to process phenylalanine.

In addition to supplying the raw material for dopamine, norepinephrine, and epinephrine, Tyrosine is used by the thyroid gland to produce thyroxine, a hormone that is involved in most body processes, helping to regulate growth rate and metabolism. A deficiency of Tyrosine can lead to hypothyroidism (low thyroid function), and Tyrosine supplements have been used to correct the problem. Tyrosine is also associated with the production of melanin, the pigmenting substance that protects the skin from harmful ultraviolet rays.

Infants with a rare genetic disorder known as tyrosinemia have difficulty processing Tyrosine. Unless intake of Tyrosine and phenylalanine is carefully restricted, this condition can lead to mental retardation.

Avoid if . . .
Due to its potential effects on the brain, it's best to avoid Tyrosine if you have a psychotic disorder. Do not give it to children.

Special Cautions
Because of its stimulative effect on the nervous system, Tyrosine can sometimes boost blood pressure or trigger anxiety and insomnia. Use it with caution if you have high blood pressure.

Possible Drug Interactions
Do not use Tyrosine if you are taking a drug classified as a monoamine oxidase (MAO) inhibitor, such as the antidepressant medications Nardil and Parnate. The combination can cause a life-threatening rise in blood pressure.

Special Information if You Are Pregnant or Breast-feeding
Do not take Tyrosine during pregnancy or breast-feeding.

Available Preparations and Dosage
Tyrosine is available in capsules and tablets in strengths of 100 to 500 milligrams. It is also available in powder form, and can be found in a variety of natural supplement preparations containing other amino acids, vitamins, and minerals. Always be careful to choose a quality brand, as some may contain impurities that could have adverse effects.

Manufacturers typically recommend dosages of 500 to 1,000 milligrams daily, taken between meals for maximum effect, or in the morning if the supplement tends to give you insomnia. Doses as high as 2,000 to 4,000 milligrams three times daily have been used to treat depression, but experts warn that you need regular monitoring by your doctor when you take doses that high.

Overdosage
Even a massive single dose is unlikely to cause harm, though it could lead to nausea and diarrhea. Sustained megadosing could theoretically strain the liver and kidneys.

Vinpocetine

Why People Take It

A so-called smart drug, Vinpocetine is said to improve memory and mental function in healthy people, as well as in those with some degree of brain impairment. Users, noting that use of the agent causes the brain to burn more oxygen and blood sugar, suggest that Vinpocetine revs up the mind. Further evidence of Vinpocetine's effect, according to advocates, is an increase in the level of adenosine triphosphate found in the brain. Adenosine triphosphate, commonly known as ATP, serves as the body's principal storehouse of ready energy.

Additional benefits attributed to Vinpocetine include an ability to relax blood vessels in the brain, thus improving circulation, and the capacity to alter blood cells so that they will be less likely to form dangerous clots. Vinpocetine has also been described as a possible antioxidant, protecting cells from the damaging free radicals that can oxidize tissues throughout the body, including the brain.

Vinpocetine is sold as a drug in Germany, Japan, Mexico, and Portugal for the treatment of cerebrovascular disorders—ailments that interrupt blood circula-

tion in the brain, starving it of oxygen. In Portugal, it's also used to treat general circulatory problems, as well as certain disorders of the eyes and ears. The drug is approved in Australia for the treatment of mental function disorders in the elderly and for other disorders of the brain. However, in the United States it remains an unapproved, experimental agent.

What It Is; How It Works
Like other members of the vinca alkaloid family of drugs, such as the cancer drugs vincristine, vinblastine, and vinorelbine, Vinpocetine comes from the periwinkle plant. Limited research data show that Vinpocetine does in fact relax the blood vessels of the brain, improve cerebral blood flow, and inhibit blood clotting to some extent. One study implies that the drug improves memory in healthy people. Studies in animals also indicate a protective effect when the brain is deprived of oxygen.

On the other hand, a number of trials have produced less encouraging results. To date, studies in people with Alzheimer's disease or stroke have been very disappointing. Trials in people with brain dysfunction due to other causes have produced mixed results, providing no clear answers for researchers. It's evident that additional, widescale studies are needed before any firm conclusions can be drawn about Vinpocetine's real value and most appropriate uses.

Avoid if . . .
Do not take Vinpocetine if you have ever had an allergic reaction to one of the vinca-based anticancer drugs, or to Vinpocetine itself.

Special Cautions

If you have liver disease, a seizure disorder, or a psychotic illness, do not take Vinpocetine except under a physician's supervision. In fact, it's a good idea to get periodic checkups while taking Vinpocetine whatever the status of your health. Your doctor will probably want to check your blood pressure on a regular basis. He or she may also want to order a routine blood test from time to time to ensure that your liver is breaking down the drug properly. Don't forget that outside the United States Vinpocetine is used like a potent prescription drug. A bit of extra caution is merited.

Side effects are relatively mild. People enrolled in research studies have taken up to 60 milligrams of Vinpocetine per day without suffering serious adverse reactions. Some people found that their blood pressure dropped slightly—an effect that can cause dizziness. Facial flushing has also occurred among people taking Vinpocetine. Other complaints reported include temporary sleep disturbances and restlessness (usually after ten weeks of therapy), pressure headache, and stomach disturbances. Minor decreases in blood sugar have been noted, too, but it has not been determined whether this effect was actually caused by Vinpocetine.

Possible Drug Interactions

Small changes in clotting time have been reported in people who combine the blood thinner Coumadin with Vinpocetine. If you are taking any type of blood thinner, be sure to let your doctor know when you begin taking Vinpocetine. While the combination does not seem to

pose a great danger, more frequent monitoring of your clotting time is a good idea.

Special Information if You Are Pregnant or Breast-feeding
During pregnancy and breast-feeding it's best to avoid any medication that's not absolutely necessary for your short-term health. Forgo Vinpocetine throughout this period.

Available Preparations and Dosage
Vinpocetine is typically sold as 5-milligram tablets. Depending on the product you purchase, the label may direct you to take anywhere from 5 to 30 milligrams daily. Do not exceed the recommended amount.

Overdosage
No information on overdosage is available.

Wheat Germ

Why People Take It
Rich in vitamins, minerals, and a unique ingredient called octacosanol, Wheat Germ is often taken to improve energy and endurance. Proponents make other claims for it as well. They say that the octacosanol in

Wheat Germ acts as a blood thinner, discouraging the formation of clots on artery walls and thus reducing the risk of a heart attack. Some experts speculate that octaconasol may also prove useful in the treatment of muscular dystrophy and other degenerative diseases of the nervous system.

Thanks to its high vitamin content, Wheat Germ also supports a healthy immune system and may help to control high cholesterol levels. And applied to the skin, wheat germ oil is used to soothe burns and sores and alleviate such skin conditions as psoriasis, seborrheic dermatitis, and abnormally dry skin.

What It Is; How It Works

Wheat Germ is the embryo of the wheat plant. In addition to octacosanol, it contains a multitude of vitamins and minerals, including calcium, copper, manganese, magnesium, most B vitamins, and phosphorus; and it's one of the richest natural sources of vitamin E. It is to these vitamins and minerals that Wheat Germ owes much of its effect.

Vitamin E, for example, is a leading antioxidant, protecting cells from destructive oxidation and possibly moderating some of the damage that occurs with age. It is also necessary for efficient immune function and the production of normal red blood cells, and it aids in controlling glucose and fat in the blood. The B vitamins play a vital role in the body's production of energy, while also supporting healthy neuromuscular function, proper digestion, normal immune function, acceptable cholesterol levels, and healthy skin, hair, and eyes. Wheat Germ is also a good source of folic acid, the vitamin that's recom-

mended during pregnancy to prevent neural tube defects from developing in the baby.

It's reasonable to suppose that the cornucopia of nutrients in Wheat Germ would have beneficial effects on energy and stamina, and several small clinical trials seem to confirm this. In particular, high-potency wheat germ oil and pure octaconasol outscored dummy medicines by as much as 100 percent in a test of their ability to boost energy and endurance.

Avoid if . . .
Wheat Germ is generally considered safe and nontoxic.

Special Cautions
Wheat Germ contains a plant-based analog of the female sex hormone estrogen; long-term use of massive doses of the high-potency oil has been known to cause testicular degeneration and loss of sex drive in some men.

Possible Drug Interactions
No drug interactions are known.

Special Information if You Are Pregnant or Breast-feeding
Some studies suggest that wheat germ oil may actually reduce the risk of miscarriage and prematurity when taken during pregnancy. Nevertheless, be sure to check with your doctor before using it, and avoid excessive doses.

Available Preparations and Dosage
Wheat Germ is available in food and as flakes to mix with food. It should be kept cool and dry, but not frozen. Wheat

germ oil can be purchased in capsule or liquid form; it should be stored tightly covered in the refrigerator.

No official dosage has been established. One to one and a half teaspoonfuls of the oil daily is often considered sufficient. Follow the manufacturer's directions whenever available.

Overdosage
No information on overdosage is available.

Whey

Why People Take It
Forget about Miss Muffet. Today, you're more likely to find *bodybuilders* eating their Whey. This milk-based supplement has recently gained popularity among athletes and fitness enthusiasts because of its rich supply of branched-chain amino acids (see separate entry). These building blocks of protein support normal growth and are said to enhance muscle mass. Whey is, in fact, a good source of a variety of proteins, and contains a minimum of unwanted fat. There's little evidence, however, that it builds muscle better than any other food rich in protein.

Most of the health claims made for Whey are based on its protein content. Proponents say that it helps to slow

aging and prevent cataracts and age-related macular degeneration. Whey and its proteins are also recommended by natural health advocates to improve appetite in cancer patients, to protect women against breast cancer, and to fight immune system diseases such as AIDS. Whey proteins have been credited with slowing the wasting effects of amyotrophic lateral sclerosis (Lou Gehrig's disease), though this disorder originates in the nervous system rather than muscle tissue. Whey is also advertised as an aid to mental alertness, memory, and sleep.

Since Whey is sold as a natural food supplement, it has undergone little medical testing, and there is scant clinical evidence to support any claimed effects beyond those that could be expected from proteins in general. Its high-protein, low-fat nutritional profile is thought to aid in weight control. An Australian study suggested that it might speed up wound healing. It has also been studied as a treatment for muscular dystrophy, but was found ineffective.

What It Is; How It Works

Whey is typically a by-product of cheese production—the substance left when the curds used to make the cheese are removed. Like most cheeses, Whey usually comes from cow's milk. In liquid form, it has long been a dietary staple wherever milk and cheese are consumed. Today, it's an ingredient in many frozen and canned prepared foods.

Whey's popularity as a powdered food supplement is relatively new. It is known to contain most of the proteins the body needs, and some preparations include additional proteins, vitamins, and minerals. Many Whey

supplements are now advertised as "ion-exchanged" or "hydrolized." Ion-exchange is a process used to remove fat and lactose, and hydrolization breaks up some proteins for better digestion.

Although the proteins in Whey are available in most ordinary diets, some researchers think that they're absorbed more quickly from Whey than from other sources. (Hence the claim that Whey is more beneficial to athletes after a workout.) The substances contained in Whey include natural growth factors, which may account for any muscle-building or wound-healing properties it exhibits. Whey also contains antioxidant compounds, providing the basis for claims that it may combat the chemical breakdowns that contribute to aging and age-related conditions such as cataracts and macular degeneration.

Avoid if . . .
People with lactose intolerance or an allergy to cows' milk should avoid Whey products.

Special Cautions
Like any type of protein, Whey can put damaging stress on the kidneys and liver when taken in massive amounts for an extended period of time.

Possible Drug Interactions
There are no known drug interactions.

Special Information if You Are Pregnant or Breast-feeding
Whey has no known harmful effects. However, be sure to check product labels for other—possibly harmful—

ingredients, and check with your doctor if you have any doubts.

Available Preparations and Dosage

Whey supplements are available in powder form, either flavored or plain, and sometimes sweetened. Many manufacturers recommend about a tablespoonful mixed with water, juice, or milk. However, ingredients and processing methods vary widely, and some brands may be purer and more effective than others.

Overdosage

As a natural substance, Whey is considered generally safe.

Usage Index

For each disease, condition, or objective listed below, this index presents the nutritional supplements that are generally considered most likely to have a positive effect. A substance is listed only if clinical research has produced encouraging results or the product's widespread acceptance suggests some satisfaction with its performance. If a claim remains speculative or theoretical, it is not included here.

Adrenal Insufficiency
DHEA

Aging
Arginine
Arginine
  Pyroglutamate
DHEA

Alcohol Withdrawal
Glutamine
Glycine

Alzheimer's Disease
Carnitine
CDP-Choline

Choline
NADH
PS
SAMe

Angina
Phosphatidylcholine

Anxiety
GABA
Inositol
PS
Tryptophan

Attention Deficit Disorder
DMAE